THE HISTORY OF MEDICINE
IN BUTLER COUNTY

By Jean B. Purvis

Heritage Publishers, Inc.

The History of Medicine in Butler County

Written by Jean B. Purvis
Edited by Karla Olson
Designed by InSync Graphic Studio

Published by
Heritage Publishers, Inc.
5312 N. Twelfth Street, Suite 302
Phoenix, Arizona 85014-2903
(602) 277-4780 (800) 972-8507

ISBN 0-929690-52-4
Library of Congress Cataloging Number 00-134177

Printed and bound in the United States of America

Contents

Foreword

The United States is unique in the world of nations in the number, diversity, and depth of commitment of its volunteers and volunteer organizations. Perhaps this was the natural result of pioneer existence; with no established network of government on the frontier, there were no organized sources of help, and families had to depend on each other in times of trouble, sickness, and tragedy.

It is logical that what started with people helping each other should become people organizing to help others. Today in the United States this helping others has been raised to the ultimate, with volunteer agencies, support groups, and United Ways to supply assistance for almost every problem that besets us.

Even in a nation of volunteers, however, Butler stands out as the archetype of the volunteer-oriented, caring community. And so it is not surprising that a prime example should be Butler Memorial Hospital. At a time when, in most communities, churches or other professional groups took the lead in establishing hospitals, in Butler the hospital was founded as a "public charity" by a group of women concerned for the poor and for the strangers in their midst.

The history of Butler Memorial Hospital, as well as other health-care services in Butler County, underlines the inspiring fact that, when a need arose, members of the community organized to provide for it. The result: hundreds of thousands of volunteers—both in the hospital and in a variety of other community agencies—have, through the years, given hundreds of thousands of hours of service.

It is indeed a wonderful, caring legacy.

PREFACE

Preparing this history of healthcare delivery in Butler County has been an exciting, frustrating, and fascinating experience. It has been a wonderful reward to discover the strong seam of caring for others that has always been an essential ingredient in what makes Butler County special. I have tried to pay tribute to those who have helped to make our community a wonderful place to live, to work, and to raise a family. This sense of community is what makes Butler special—and what I have learned is that it has always been this way.

I apologize in advance for any omissions; they were inadvertent. Sometimes references were not available. The pressures of space and time and economics have also operated to limit the inclusion of stories and details.

I wish I could list everyone who helped in the task of reconstructing the way things were and how they have evolved, but that would be impossible. Many of those who generously took time from their busy lives to share their memories and experiences with me have been quoted directly; but there were so many others who contributed valuable information that if I named them all it would make another book.

I am especially grateful to the following, whose generosity went beyond what I had a right to expect:

Eileen Morrow, whose treasure trove of clippings, pictures, and information about the history of the nurses' training school and the nursing association, were invaluable.

Carol Osgood, who shared a wealth of informative hospital publications and memories.

Mary Wilson Sage, who provided me with valuable resources on the 1918 flu pandemic.

LeRoy Kuhn, whose wonderful reminiscences provided color to the picture of medicine in the twenties, and whose memories of the Easter Seal Society were especially valuable.

The Butler Public Library, in particular LuAnne Eisler in the Genealogy Room, who helped me research old newspapers, cemetery lists, obituaries, and other valuable sources of information; and Joe Yerace, who helped me run the microfilm machines and print articles I needed.

The Butler County Historical Society, for allowing me to borrow early histories, as well as providing information from early newspapers.

Louise Hetrick, volunteer par excellence, whose hours spent working for the hospital in the auxiliary add up to thousands.

Mary Hulton Phillips, also an auxilian, but perhaps better known for her leadership in the March of Dimes;

those who marched remember that it always seemed to take place on a January night that was either wet or snowy, but somehow was always successful.

All those who shared their memories of the 1918 flu in Butler. I wish I could have included all of them.

Joe Randig, who provided a wonderful first-hand account of the terror of polio in the late forties and early fifties.

Lucille Swigart, Martha McGinley, Ann McCarren, and Faye Silverio, now retired, who took time to describe what nursing was like when they were newly "capped" and how it has changed through the years.

The Butler County Medical Society, both the organization and individual members who took time to talk with me. The minutes of meetings in the twenties, thirties, and fifties were a great help in recreating the medical concerns of the period.

The Butler Eagle, for permitting me to go through their files for articles and photographs—and, specifically, Mark Mann, Dave Heastings, and Kelly Garrett.

And so many others, I cannot name them all. Any small virtues of the book belong to you; any deficits are mine alone.

My special gratitude to John Righetti and BMH for giving me this project. I have learned so much and enjoyed it so much (in spite of complaints!) that I can't say thank you enough. ▨

Jean B. Purvis

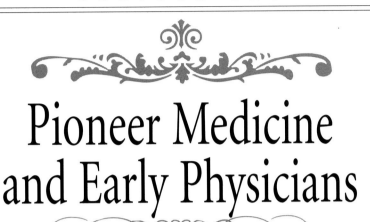

CHAPTER ONE

Pioneer Medicine and Early Physicians

Pioneer Medicine

efore 1800, the area that now makes up Butler County was primarily the hunting reserve of Seneca Indians; and a few brave settlers. Then in 1785, with the second treaty of Fort Stanwyx, the area was formally conveyed to the Commonwealth of Pennsylvania. However, even before it was officially its property, the state legislature moved to dispose of this land. In 1783, the legislature agreed to use the land to redeem the "depreciated" certificates issued to the Revolutionary War soldiers in lieu of money. The county was divided into two areas, and land in those areas was awarded to the soldiers according to rank. Ironically, the "struck" lands—those areas struck from the rolls because they were "unfit for cultivation"—proved later to contain rich oil seams.

The legislature formally created Butler County on March 12, 1800, and three years later the first lots were sold in what was to become the city of Butler. H.M. Brackenridge described the town in *Recollections of the West:* "On my arrival in Butler there were a few log houses raised, but not sufficiently completed to be occupied. It was not long before there were two taverns, a store and

a blacksmith shop, it was then a town. The county around was a howling wilderness… ." [1]

Pioneer medicine in that wilderness was basic, usually a matter of herbs and hope and folk remedies, with a little bloodletting on the side. Childhood diseases were many and often fatal. Croup, dysentery, diphtheria, scarlet fever, as well as the usual childhood ailments, all took their toll of children. Sometimes, parents lost whole families.

Gunshot and other wounds were treated with slippery elm bark, flax seed, and other poultices. For rheumatism, sufferers ap-plied the oil of rattlesnakes, geese, bears, wolves, raccoons, groundhogs, and polecats to the joints and rubbed it in before the fire. They treated *erysipelas* (a *streptococcus* infection also known as St. Anthony's Fire) with the blood of a black cat, and, according to *Pioneer Medicine in Western Pennsylvania,* most black cats had ears or tail cropped. [2] When all else failed, many turned to charms and incantations, perhaps as effective as some of the other remedies.

Housewives and midwives were the first, and often the only, source of treatment for the family, since there were few doctors. Many doctors, even if available, had little more training or knowledge than their patients. Childbirth was the business of women, attended by a midwife if available—otherwise a knowledgeable relative. A doctor was summoned in only the most difficult and desperate cases.

At this time, most doctors were without formal medical training and relied on a handful of general medical books, such as *Gunn's Domestic Medicine* or *Poor Man's Friend*. Although medical schools began to flourish in the nineteenth century, most medical education was an apprenticeship, in which an aspiring student would pay a doctor a fee (usually around $100) and agree to remain with his master for two to five years. The student's duties could range from currying the doctor's horse to compounding medicines, as well as—perhaps—helping to treat patients.

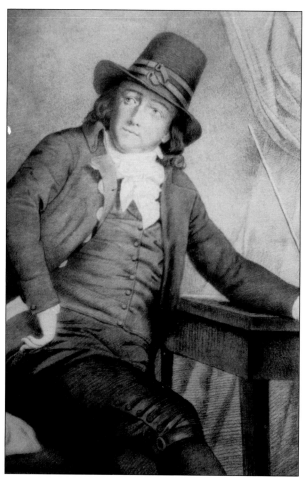

Baron Detmar Basse came from Germany in 1802 and founded Zelienople. He brought with him an extensive knowledge of drugs and herbs, which he used for the benefit of the community, and thus was given the title of doctor.

The medical schools that did exist had virtually no entrance requirements. Even by the outbreak of the Civil War there were no effective licensing laws in any state and consequently, almost anyone could call himself a doctor. Many did.

Surgery was both painful and dangerous. There were no anesthetics except alcohol and some herbs, and there was the ever-present danger of gangrene or infection. As a consequence, surgery was a last resort, confined to urgent problems: gunshot wounds, abscesses, treatment of hernias and fractures, and only the most

difficult and desperate obstetrical cases. It wasn't until 1825 that the cesarean section was performed as an operation to save *both* mother and child. Prior to that time it was performed only to deliver the child when the mother had died.

With these "givens," it is part of Butler's special quality that the early doctors here were neither charlatans nor untrained.

Early Physicians

The first "doctor" in Butler County was the Baron Detmar Basse, who came from Germany in 1802 and founded Zelienople. The first "real doctor with a medical degree" was Dr. Christoff Mueller, who came to Butler County from Germany with George Rapp, founder of the Harmony Society, in 1803. [2] The Harmonists, a German religious sect, settled in southwest Butler County on land purchased from Detmar Basse. Mueller was the first doctor in Pennsylvania north of the Ohio River. [3] He was also a trained botanist and talented musician, who was responsible for the school, the zoo, the orchestra, and the museum in the Harmony community. His botanical garden, in which he grew medicinal herbs, was "an elegant collection of plants, carefully arranged according to the Linnaean system," according to John Melish, one of the first Anglo-Americans to visit the Society in 1811.

As Shelby Ruch points out, like most other doctors of this period, Mueller believed in whisky as a medication. Recipes for tonics and cough medicines typically contained alcohol and opium. For example, Delicious Cough Syrup! called for half rye whisky and half New Orleans molasses spiked with oil of tar and balsam fir. Most people believed in taking a spring tonic, and many of these included alcohol. One local tonic called for one pint of "good brandy," a pint of cod liver oil, and a dozen fresh eggs. Another popular spring dose was sulphur and molasses. [4]

Ruch also notes that, although doctors were respected in the community, they were not above criticism. He quotes from a letter Abraham Ziegler wrote in 1848: "As respects my rheumatic pains they are not better and the medicine Mr. Shrivir presented to me done me no good. Also the vial of Peach Oil I got from Dr. Linenbrink turned out to be Caster Oil when I came to use it. You will please tell H . . . Doctor to be more careful distributing his medicine." [5]

Perhaps because it was a settled and organized community almost from the beginning, a number of well-trained physicians followed Dr. Mueller to the Harmony/ Zelienople area. Dr. Loring Lusk, who practiced in Harmony and Zelienople at various times between 1823 and 1878, had two sons who became doctors and also practiced in Harmony. Dr. Joseph Lusk, who was educated at Mercer Academy and graduated from Western Reserve Medical College in 1850,

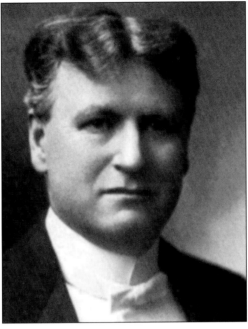

Dr. J.C. Boyle was one of Butler County's first specialists. Graduating from the Western Pennsylvania Medical College in 1892, he took graduate courses in diseases of the eye in Philadelphia and in London, England, as well as a special course in ear, nose and throat, before returning to Butler.

practiced in Harmony from that year until elected to the legislature in 1870. He served for six years then set up his practice in Butler. Dr. Amos Lusk studied with his father and opened an office in Harmony in 1849, then moved to Zelienople two years later. In 1853, he was placed in charge of the United States Marine Hospital in Pittsburgh. He stayed there four years, then moved to Missouri, returning to Zelienople in 1862. The younger Lusk was also, according to Ruch, a banker and an educator who worked to improve the schools, and he was reputed to have mastered thirty-five languages.

Dr. Mueller was followed by Dr. George Miller, son of a professor of mathematics and natural sciences at Jefferson College in Canonsburg, Pennsylvania. He studied with Dr. Letherman of that city, coming to Butler in 1814 or 1815. According to James McKee's *History of Butler County*, he was "said to have been the only physician in Butler County at the time of the agrarian troubles on the Maxwell Farm (1815). In October of that year when Maxwell was wounded, Dr. Miller came to his aid, while a messenger was sent to Pittsburgh for Dr. Agnew, who arrived that evening." [6] Maxwell was shot during an altercation between farmers and land speculators who claimed the land they occupied. The speedy arrival of Dr. Agnew from Pittsburgh is just short of amazing, given the state of transportation at the time.

Dr. Henry C. De Wolfe, a Yale graduate, came to Butler in 1817 or 1818. He was active in the commu-

LETTER TO THE BUTLER SENTINEL

Messrs, Editors: On the 28th of November last, the following extraordinary surgical operation was performed on my son: The circumstances leading to the operation were these: My son James, aged eight years, being sent for a few sticks of wood, and having to pass by a horse that was feeding, was kicked by him on the left side of his head, which fractured his scull in so shocking a manner, that some of the brain came out. The boy lay in this situation; without sense or motion for about 22 hours, while I sent for Doctor Linn, of Butler, and Doctor Holmes, of Pittsburgh.

Immediately after the surgeons arrived, they laid my son upon a table, opened the instruments, trepanned the scull, and took out the broken pieces of bone, the end of one of which had made a dent in the striffen, an inch in length, and penetrated the substance of the brain, leaving a space without bone 3 inches in length and 2 in breadth.—During the operation, a considerable quantity of the brain was lost, which flowed through the apperture in the striffen.

Much praise is due the surgeons for their skill; dexterity, and great composure, during the painful operation.

As an instrument in the hand of Providence, much credit is due Dr. Linn for his great skill, and persevering energy, in arresting the progress of inflammation and restoring my son to a complete state of health. He is now perfectly sensible, in good health, and the wound is completely healed over.

JAMES LOVE

Buffalo township, Butler co. March 22, 1825

A letter to the Sentinel describes one of Dr. Linn's challenging – and amazing – cases – Courtesy of Butler Public Library nity: a trustee of the academy; treasurer of the borough; and, according to R.C. Brown, "filled many other local offices during his long residence here." He died in 1854. His son, a graduate of Cleveland Medical College, practiced in Butler from 1851 until his untimely death in 1859 at the age of 35.

Dr. George Linn came to Butler from Mercer County in 1823. In his Recollections, published in the *Butler Sentinel*, John H. Negley says, "Dr. George Linn was one of the best and most highly esteemed physicians Butler ever had. He had a good practice, was a good man, and his death in 1833 was highly regretted." (7)

An unusual and apparently successful operation was performed by Dr. Du Panchell, a Frenchman and a "polished and learned physician," according to R.C. Brown's *History of Butler County*. Brown reports that "Patrick Kelly's Dutch hostler, whose head was not altogether 'level,' was subject to heroic treatment by Dr. Du Panchell. He [cut out pieces of] the skull with such success as to render the hostler a sensible mortal." (8)

Dr. James Graham, a native of Ireland, opened a school on McKean Street and taught there, in addition to practicing medicine.

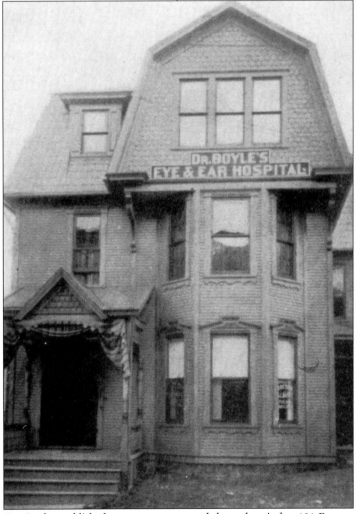

Dr. Boyle established an eye, ear, nose and throat hospital at 121 East Cunningham Street.

His methods were certainly draconian. A student wrote of him that "he brought from the old country some of the methods of school teaching. One of these was the taws, or cat-of-nine-tails, as a whip for a bad boy." Brown reports "he was a thorough physician and a scholar and in his sober hours he was popular, but the use of drink led to his death." (9)

Dr. Graham was not unusual in having an avocation other than medicine: Dr. Brower of Prospect (1838) was elected to the legislature; Dr. George Gettys (1843) had an interest in one of Butler's Whig newspapers; Dr. Lusk, who practiced first in Harmony and later Butler, was a geologist and archeologist, as well as a member of the legislature; and Dr. Sylvester Bell, who practiced first in Chicora and later in Butler, was also a member of the state legislature.

A less savory member of the profession, Dr. Henri de Coliere, was placed on trial for manslaughter for "using the knife," according to Brown. De Coliere also diagnosed a case of delirium tremens and declared the patient would die "in three minutes" and, Brown says, to make his prediction good he administered a poison that accomplished it. (10)

Probably the best known of the early physicians was Dr. A.M. Neyman, who practiced from 1851 until he retired some years before he died in 1911. He also taught before going into medicine.

Dr. Neyman's long and successful practice included several firsts: he was the first physician in Pennsylvania to take a post graduate course. Even more noteworthy, he performed a cesarean section, the first authenticated operation of its kind west of the Alleghenies. Both mother and child survived.

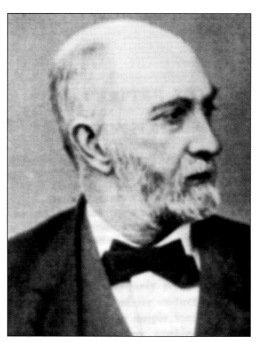

Dr. Amos Lusk was the first president of the Butler County Medical Society, organized in 1866.

On November 3, 1866, twelve doctors met and formed the Butler County Medical Society. They elected Dr. Amos Lusk, president; Dr. Neyman, vice president; Dr. S. Bredin, secretary; and Drs. McMichael, Cowden, and Lusk, censors. A committee was appointed to draft a constitution and bylaws. The minutes say that "after a pleasant interchange of sentiment, and supper of oysters served in style at the hotel table, the meeting adjourned to convene at the same place January 3, 1867."

Butler's Early Female Doctors

By the second half of the nineteenth century, Butler had well-trained practicing physicians in most of the county. In 1881, the state required physicians to register with the county in which they practiced, and that year, there were sixty-nine physicians registered in Butler County. [12]

Among those listed in 1883 is Mary E. Harper of Bald Ridge (Renfrew), the first woman doctor in Butler.

The histories give no other information. However, a Dr. E.D. Harper moved from Bakerstown to Bald Ridge in January of that year, and his family joined him in April, according to the newspapers. It is possible Dr. Mary Harper was his wife.

There is only one mention of her in the newspapers of that year. The Butler Eagle for August 1, 1883, announced:

Butler County has a doctress (sic) in the person of Mrs. Mary Harper of Bald Ridge. She registered her name and diploma as a regular practicing physician last week in the Prothonotary's office.

It was not easy for a woman to become a doctor in the nineteenth century. Medical schools did not admit women until 1849, and no hospital would take women as interns and residents until the first hospital run entirely by women was established in 1857. Nevertheless, Dr. Mary Harper was the first of a number of women physicians who practiced in Butler County.

Dr. Eliza Grossman, a graduate of Wooster Medical College in Ohio, followed in 1890. She practiced with her husband, Dr. Robert Grossman, until her death from a respiratory infection in 1896. Her obituary in The Butler Eagle called her "a highly esteemed member of the profession of her choice," and went on to say, "Having spent most of her life equipping herself for a useful and honorable career, her early demise is attended by unusual sadness." [13]

Patent Cure-Alls

In an era when there were few effective medicines or drugs, it was natural for people to want to believe in the miracles promised by patent medicines. And they did offer hope and promise miracles. In the nineteenth century, with no Food and Drug Administration to monitor them, patent medicines flourished. Dr. Townsend claimed that his compound extract of sarsaparilla "purifies the whole system and strengthens the person . . .creates new, rich, and pure blood, a power possessed by no other medicine. . .It has cured within the last five years more than 100,000 cases of severe disease; at least 15,000 were considered incurable."

Often the advertisements were a few sentences in the middle of a news column:

> *Drunkenness—Liquor Habit—In All The World There Is But One Cure. Dr. Haines Golden Specific.*

And, in the same paper:

> *I gave the child a dose of Dr. Sellers' Cough Syrup. And it was all right in an hour. Sold by druggists at 25 cents per bottle.* ⁽¹¹⁾

No patent medicine would be complete without the testimonial. Headed "A Perfect Remedy in 20 Diseases", this one had marvelous claims:

> *I am verging on eighty years and deem it my duty to suffering humanity to say that my long life is due to Brandreth's Pills, which have been my sole medicine for half a century. I know the last forty-three years of my life is owing solely to their use. Your pills saved me many times after the best medical skill in several states had given me up as hopeless. I have had many converts to purgation with Brandreth's Pills and have seen them perform almost miracles of cure. For children, a few doses have cured measles, scarlet fever and whooping cough. In all female troubles and weakness I have never known them to fail. In adult males I have known them to cure the worst cases of dyspepsia, rheumatism, kidney diseases, dysentery and diarrhea; even dropsy, paralysis and apoplexy have yielded to a persistent course of Brandreth's Pills. In fact, I have found them to be the true Life Elixir. They act as continual preventives against the effects of time, disease, and labor.*

With this miracle cure available, it's a wonder anyone died!

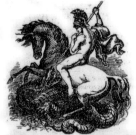

HOSTETTER'S CELEBRATED STOMACH BITTERS.

A pure and powerful Tonic, corrective and alterative of wonderful efficacy in disease of the

Stomach, Liver and Bowels.

Cures Dyspepsia, Liver Complaint, Headache, General Debility, Nervousness, Depression of Spirits, Constipation, Colic, Intermittent Fevers, Cramps and Spasms, and all Complaints of either Sex, arising from Bodily Weakness whether inherent in the system or produced by special causes.

NOTHING that is not wholesome, genial and restorative in its nature enters into the composition of HOSTETTER'S STOMACH BITTERS.

A typical patent medicine advertisement

A typical patent medicine advertisement of the 19th century.   Courtesy of Butler Public Library

Her sister, Dr. Louisa Shryock, also graduated from Wooster, as well as "West Penn Medical College of Pittsburg." She practiced in her brother-in-law's office until tuberculosis forced her to retire several years before her death in 1903. Both sisters were members of the Butler County Medical Society, obviously a much more progressive group than the American Medical Association, which did not admit women until 1915.

A number of other female physicians followed; some, like Dr. Eliza Grossman, practiced with their husbands.

Homeopaths and Osteopaths

The first homeopathic physician in the county was Dr. P.S. Duff. In 1863, according to McKee, "he was a man of education, a successful physician and a useful citizen." Other homeopaths included Dr. William H. Brown, who located here in 1893 and practiced until May 1904, when he retired because of his health. He was one of the doctors who "did noble work in Butler during the winter of 1903 and 1904, made memorable by the typhoid epidemic. The exposure of the winter brought on a fatal disease that caused his death in June 1905." [14]

The first osteopathic physician came to Butler in 1901. Dr. William Smith, a graduate of a medical college in Scotland, became interested in osteopathy and taught in the first school of osteopathy in Kirksville, Missouri. He remained in Butler only a few months, returning to Missouri to teach, but he was followed by many others. Dr. E.H. Merkley, who came to Butler in 1901 after Dr. Smith left, was "the real pioneer osteopath of Butler." [15] He sold his practice to Dr. Julia Foster in 1902. She was eventually joined by her son, Dr. J.C. Foster.

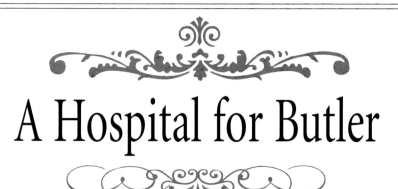

A Hospital for Butler

The Ladies' Hospital Association

In the summer of 1896 several tragic events occurred in the Butler County community. First, two young men, strangers, one from Kentucky and one from Ohio, died from fever. Since they were from out of state, they had no families to care for them during their illnesses. Next, several train wrecks highlighted the lack of emergency care in the community. A group of prominent, civic-minded women determined that something must be done to care for the indigent, the sick and injured.

Three of the women, Elizabeth McCandless, Harriet Cooper, and Mrs. T.J. Steen, wrote a letter to Andrew

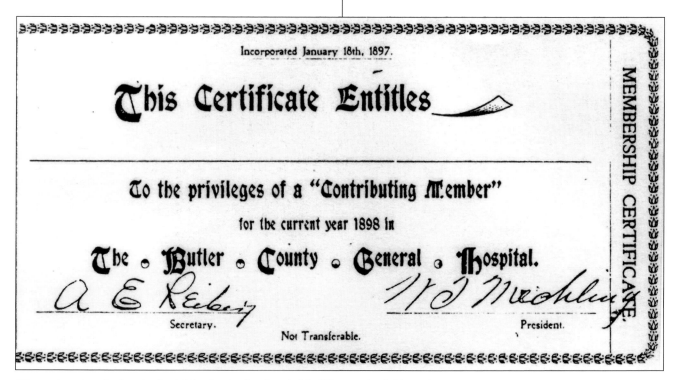

Those who subscribed to the fund drive for the first hospital building received this receipt.

Carnegie requesting his help. Although his charitable gifts were chiefly to libraries and educational institutions, Carnegie promised them $1,500 for the building of a hospital once the community showed good faith by coming up with an organization and some funds.

Wasting no time, the women called a meeting for November 17, 1897, held in the YMCA building in Butler. About eighty women, representing all the churches and the women's societies in Butler, showed up. Mrs. M.S. Templeton, Mrs. J.B. Black, and Mrs. W.C. Thompson were appointed to prepare a constitution and bylaws and present them at the next meeting, which was scheduled for the following week. At that meeting, they

elected officers, appointed a finance committee, and elected a board of management, consisting of two representatives from each of the churches in town. They called their group the Ladies' Hospital Association.

In January, they announced their fund-raising plans. "A committee has been appointed for each ward and a thorough canvassing of the town will be made. It is hoped that every citizen will respond liberally and promptly when called upon by the ladies." [17] The Ladies' Hospital Association and the advisory board they had selected—L.O. Purvis; John S. Campbell; Alfred Wick; Joseph Hartman; J.M. Galbreath; W.T. Mechling; Dr. A.M. Neyman; L.R. Schmerz, and Daniel Younkins—as

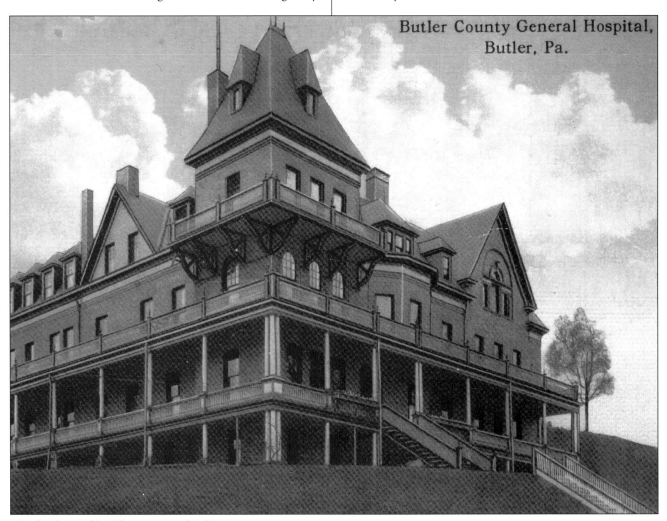

Butler County General Hospital, Butler, Pa.

The first hospital building was completed in 1898.   Courtesy of Butler Memorial Hospital

The Hospital's First Mission Statement and First Annual Report

The Centennial Souvenir booklet, *published in 1900, described the work of the hospital association this way:*

> *The object of the association is the maintenance of a general hospital as a public charity. It is intended and designed for accident and emergency cases, cases of sudden attack and sickness where patients have no immediate friends or homes for their care and provision. No worthy charity cases are refused. . . . The hospital is dependent upon public benevolence and the receipts from pay[ing] patients for its maintenance, being assisted by a small apportionment from the state for that purpose. It is nonsectarian in its management, the charter providing that no more than two of the directors be from the same church organization, and no one shall be excluded from its privileges by reason of race, religious beliefs or distinctions.*
>
> *The capacity of the hospital is twenty-two persons. They employ a superintendent, three nurses, cook, laundress and janitor. . . .*
>
> *Another organization exists within the hospital proper as a permanent auxiliary to the same called "The Ladies' Hospital Association.". . . To them are due all the careful appointments of the hospital, and they are entrusted with the details of the work. The rates for the hospital for patients, including boarding, laundry and medicine are as follows: Wards, $7 per week; private rooms, $10 and $15 per week. The hospital always has the care of a large number of patients. It is now in a first-class condition, and has deservedly won the confidence and generous support of the people of this county.* [18]

The hospital's first annual report, issued in 1900, lists the following:

Receipts $4,517.20
    Receipts from patients $3,076.90
    Receipts from county and boro $190.30
    Receipts from State of Pa $1,250.00
Expenses for 1900 $5,594.73

Other statistics provide the reason for the deficit; of 148 patients admitted, 52 were charity patients, accounting for about one-sixth of the patient days.

well as others interested in the project, set out to "maintain a general hospital as a public charity at Butler, Pennsylvania, to be known as 'The Butler County General Hospital.'"

Fund-raising was so successful that it attracted the attention of Thomas Robinson, who had apparently applied for a charter for a hospital some years before. He wrote a letter to *The Butler County Herald* complaining about the women's efforts. The women knew nothing of Robinson's efforts, but promptly appointed a committee to meet with a committee of his organization. At this meeting they determined that Robinson's

group had nothing but a charter. Members of Robinson's group admitted that they had no site, no subscriptions, and that they believed that the organization had ceased to exist. When the president of the Ladies' Association asked, "If we retire now and give the old association a clear field, will you take up the work and carry it through to a successful issue?" all the members of the former group responded, "We bid you Godspeed in this noble work."

Encouraged, the Ladies' Hospital Association secured a site from the John Muntz estate south of Connoquenessing Creek at the foot of Main Street.

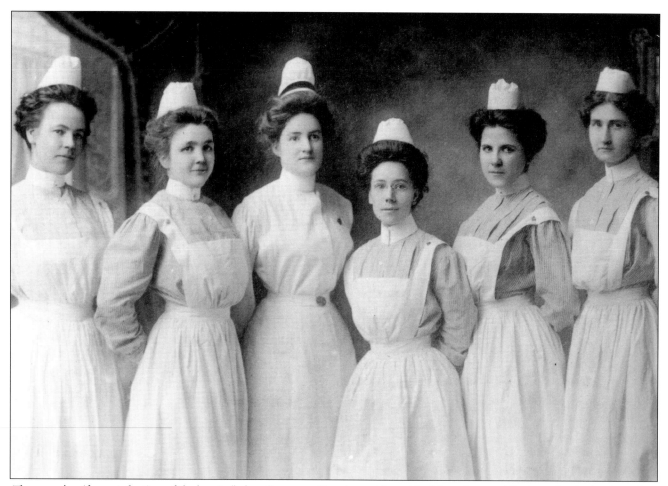

The nurses' uniform at the time of the hospital's founding was a blue dress with a white bib and apron. The hem, four inches from the floor, barely hid black cotton stockings and black oxfords. The tour of duty was 12 hours daily, with one afternoon off per week— although extra time was granted to attend church. All recitations were given before noon, and all doctors' lectures were after 7 p.m.
Courtesy of Butler Memorial Hospital Nurses' Alumnae Association

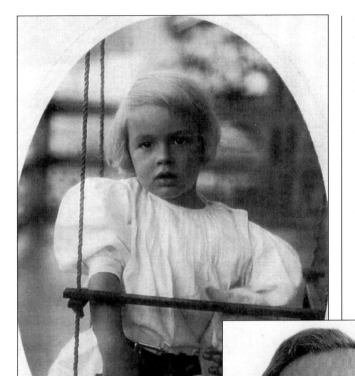

Edwin Howard as a four-year-old child and as a man. He was the first baby to be born in Butler Hospital. Mrs. George Howard, the 1372nd patient, was admitted with a diagnosis of pregnancy and delivered of a son October 28, 1904. Edwin Howard became an architect. This was a time when women had their babies at home—another would not be born in the hospital until two years later and it was several years before very many were born there.

Courtesy of Edwin Howard

They developed plans for a building with twenty-one bedrooms. Bids were opened July 29, with construction to begin immediately and be finished by the following winter.

Not surprisingly, this was too optimistic. It was not until June of the following year that the Ladies' Hospital Association invited the public to an "old-fashioned house warming," a program of music and speeches; "contributions in the form of cash or donations of groceries, canned fruit, general house furnishing articles are earnestly solicited." In a word, those attending this "house warming" were encouraged to give anything they could. Due to the extraordinary efforts of the women's organization and the Butler County community, everything they needed was acquired. The building had cost $25,000, and Andrew Carnegie made good on his offer of $1,500 toward the cost.

For several years, the hospital was maintained *solely* by community support and donations of food, hospital gowns, and all the daily necessities. The Ladies' Hospital Association sewed tirelessly to supply sheets, pillowcases, gowns, towels, uniforms, and other needs. Families donated blankets and quilts. The women put on benefit plays, asked for contributions, and gave their time and money generously.

On July 6, 1899, the hospital opened its doors to its first patient—a thirty-five-year-old man from Poughkeepsie, New York, with a crushed foot. Doctors operated on him twice and he was finally discharged in April, after a 278-day stay. Doctors treated another man for a sprained foot. On July 17, a twenty-nine-year-old man, described as from Italy with three years in this country, was admitted with a broken leg and stayed one day short of a month.

All told, the hospital had six patients that first July. They treated forty patients during the first half year, dealing with a variety of problems: fractures, malaria, "organic heart trouble," "exhaustion from exposure and hunger," rheumatism, seven cases of typhoid fever (one died), and a railway accident.

Clearly the hospital was fulfilling its mission.

Twenty-three of the patients were from Butler County. Others were from nearby—Warren, Clarion, Pittsburgh; some were from farther away—Ontario, England, Italy, Ireland, Germany. One was listed as having "no residence."

During the first full year of operation the hospital cared for a grand total of ninety-four patients, and the second year 144, with thirteen cases of typhoid that year. Already there was some international diversity: five Austrians, eleven Germans, six Italians, five Irish, and one Assyrian. The remarks line in the hospital record often included the patient's religion (one was listed as an infidel) and marital status, as well as friends or relatives.

The Nurses Training School

When the hospital was first opened, the superintendent and helpers from the community cared for the patients, but most helpers did not stay long. The superintendent instructed the helpers while her assistant was in charge of the operating room and the kitchen and was on night call for emergencies. Clearly this arrangement was not satisfactory as the hospital grew. The need for trained staff was apparent.

In 1901, Butler Hospital established the nurses training school, to provide skilled nurses to care for the growing number of patients. [19] It graduated its first class in 1903.

The Ladies' Hospital Association held a banquet for the two young graduates. The graduation ceremony itself must have seemed almost as long as the training; there were vocal and piano solos, and an address given by the Reverend Maitland Alexander, pastor of the First Presbyterian Church of Pittsburgh and president of Allegheny General Hospital. Another solo, and then Dr. J.C. Boyle of the hospital staff spoke to the nurses. He told the audience that the hospital staff was sure that they would "reflect credit on their profession and their Alma Mater."

A.E. Reiber presented the diplomas and badges to the graduates. In a short talk he reviewed the history and work of the hospital and the training school, commenting that eight students were taking the course (including the two who had just completed it). He concluded by saying, "Since the (Butler Hospital) was opened five years ago, it has cared for 1,045 patients, many of whom were charity patients." [20]

None of the participants in the ceremony realized that the hospital and the town were about to encounter their gravest crisis so far—the typhoid epidemic of 1903–1904.

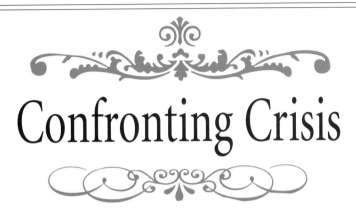

CHAPTER THREE

Confronting Crisis

Typhoid

yphoid fever had been prevalent since people began to live in larger settlements and share sources of water. It is caused by a bacterium shed in the urine and feces of infected people, or by flies traveling from feces to food, or by food handlers who are carriers of the disease. Consequently, water supplies in residential areas where there was no sewage system were easily contaminated. Symptoms of the disease, which usually begin gradually eight to fourteen days after infection, include fever, headache, joint pain, sore throat, constipation or diarrhea, loss of appetite, and abdominal pain and tenderness. Today, with antibiotic treatment, more than 99 percent of typhoid cases are cured. Before antibiotics, however, there were more than 30 deaths per 100,000 population in the United States alone. (1900 statistic) [21]

In late October 1903, forty-seven people in Butler County sickened, but it appears no one was really worried. The doctors weren't even sure the afflicted had typhoid. Early November, however, brought so many cases—four in the hospital the first week alone—that the local Board of Health began to investigate. An article in *The Butler Eagle* on November 7 explained that:

> Up to the first of October, nearly every case of fever in Butler had come from abroad, [in this context "abroad" and "foreign" mean out of the county] but at the present time the majority of cases can be assigned to no foreign cause and the members of the Board of Health have decided to find out if there are any local causes for the outbreak or whether it can only be attributed to the season of the year, which among physicians is generally known as the "fall typhoid season," and to the fact that it is generally prevalent throughout the country. [22]

No one knew exactly how many cases there were in the borough of Butler, but there were nine cases at the hospital, and a number of doctors reported one to three cases each being cared for at home. Two people had died.

COMMONWEALTH OF PENNSYLVANIA.
DEPARTMENT OF HEALTH

TYPHUS FEVER!

THESE PREMISES ARE UNDER STATE QUARANTINE.

No person shall be permitted to enter, leave, or take any article from this house without written permission from a legally authorized agent of the State Department of Health, excepting physicians and trained nurses in charge of the sick.

Animals must not be permitted to leave these premises.

No person other than those authorized by the Department of Health shall remove this placard. Any person or persons defacing, covering up, or destroying this placard render themselves liable to the penalties of the law.

"Act of Assembly approved May 28, 1915, provides that anyone violating the provisions of this Act, upon conviction thereof may be sentenced to pay a fine of not less than $10.00 or more than $100.00, to be paid to the use of said county, and costs of prosecution, or to be imprisoned in the county jail for a period of not less than ten days or more than thirty days, or both, at the discretion of the court."

By order of the Department of Health,

SAMUEL G. DIXON, M. D.,
Commissioner of Health.

....
Health Officer.

....
Address.

Posted .... 191...

Typhoid Quarantine sign used by the city of Butler   Courtesy of the City of Butler

Investigators did not believe that the local water supply was the problem, since the water came from the new Thorn Run Dam. However, they eventually determined that the water was indeed contaminated. Apparently the filter beds had been out of commission for a few days and the water, contaminated by sewage from farm houses where there were a number of cases of typhoid, had poured into the dam unfiltered.

By the end of November there were 976 cases. During the worst of the epidemic, 710 cases were reported in 72 hours. A canvass of the town showed that at least one house in every five had from one to five cases. Officials closed the schools, and doctors worked around the clock but could not take care of everybody.

The town organized a relief society, and the state board sent Dr. Wilbur R. Batt, quarantine officer at large, to help the local board. He established a dispensary in the Duffy building on the corner of Main and Jefferson streets, where a skilled nurse kept a complete supply of disinfectants and chemicals and explained how to use them. Six temporary hospitals were set up and in operation from December 1 to March 1. These hospitals treated forty typhoid patients.

Meanwhile, Butler Hospital opened its doors to the afflicted, treating sixty-nine patients from December 1 to January 1, forty-nine of them free of charge. A group of Butler County residents, led by Dr. Robert Greer, raised more than $65,000 for relief.

McKee's description of the epidemic was obviously written from first-hand experience. It vividly recounts a town in panic, mustering every resource. Help flowed in from neighboring towns, which sent generous contributions to the relief fund; in addition, physicians and nurses volunteered their services and worked long hours without charge. [23]

The ladies' auxiliary to the relief committee made it their business to visit every stricken home, to provide necessities and help look after children. Contributions poured in before Christmas, including an enormous box of dolls from a wholesaler in Pittsburgh, and by Christmas Eve the committee was able to provide a present for every sick child, as well as to others whose families could not provide them.

Clara Barton, who had organized the United States branch of the Red Cross in 1881-82 and served as its president until 1904, came to Butler in December of 1903 to help with the typhoid epidemic. She and her staff made a through examination of the hospitals, diet kitchen, supply department and method of conducting relief work. They were pleased to find that the way the relief work had been organized was equal to other places where the National Red cross had taken charge.

Final count of the typhoid epidemic (called by many the worst epidemic Butler has ever seen) was 1,587 cases of the fever, with 127 deaths. The hospital had cared for 153 cases.

Beyond Typhoid

Typhoid would remain endemic for some years. In 1912, for example, there were twenty-one cases between July and December. (Many of those, however, originated "abroad".) In 1919, there was another scare when thirty cases were announced. But by 1923, the minutes of the Butler County Medical Society stated that "typhoid is now a rare disease."

Other diseases were prevalent, however. City health records for the period show cases of diphtheria, scarlet fever, and measles, all contagious diseases that required a quarantine sign posted on the patient's house. In addition, in July 1900, *The Millerstown Herald* reported a case of smallpox in Butler Township. The family was quarantined and the state board of health ordered vaccinations for all who had been exposed and for all unvaccinated school children. In spite of these precautions, there were enough cases that in 1903 the city set up a smallpox hospital in a house so patients could be isolated and treated. [29]

The smallpox hospital remained in operation, off and on until at least August 1907, when the report for the preceding month reads "Visits to smallpox hospital—4."

Industry and Immigration

Industry Comes to Butler

The original admission books of Butler County General Hospital give a vivid picture of the waves of immigrants that came in response to the founding of the Standard Steel Car plant in Lyndora. There were plenty of opportunities for men and women who were willing to work. In 1902, the records show there were thirty-nine Italian, three French, six German, and six Austrian admissions to the hospital. By 1903, there was another increase, and it reflects the wave of immigration from eastern Europe: fifteen Greeks, fifteen Poles, and thirty-two Slavs, as well as assorted western Europeans and a few Scandinavians.

The hospital needed more beds, and in 1904 they built a two-story brick addition. The first floor was used as a laundry and the second floor as living apartments for the help, leaving all of the original space for expanding patient care.

In 1906, nineteen members of the hospital staff formed the Nurses Alumnae Association. The administration lengthened the nurses training program to

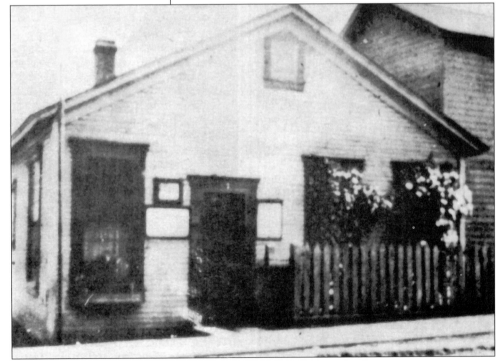

The little "Red Row" building that served as Anna Brown's office was provided by Standard Steel. One of its popular features was a bathtub that anyone could use, provided he brought his own towel and soap and left the tub spotless for the next bather. Courtesy of Bruce Stamm and Pullman Standard

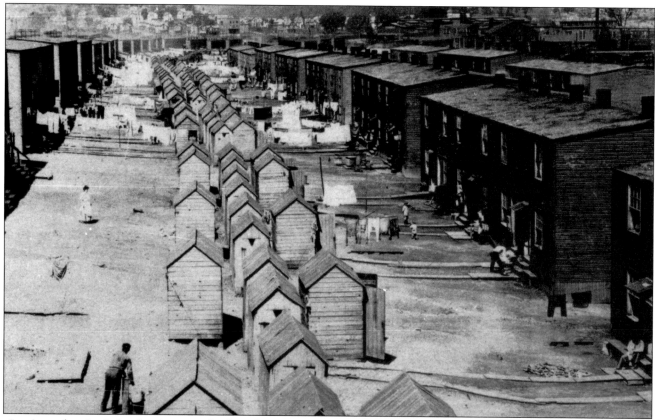

Immigrant housing in Lyndora known as "Red Row." Courtesy of Pullman Standard

three years and added bacteriology, gynecology, cooking and surgery to the curriculum for the eleven students.

From this time on hospital records show a number of industrial accidents. Often the home address is given as "Red Row," or "Company Shanty" or "RR Shanty." This was the immigrant housing in Lyndora, so called because the rows of houses had been literally painted red.

On October 6, 1907, Butler experienced its greatest industrial accident. An explosion of molten metal at the Standard Steel plant injured at least sixty men, many seriously. Seventeen died. Every passing vehicle helped transport the injured to the hospital. Fifty-seven were admitted, and there were not enough beds for them all. "Many dozens of cots were brought in from furniture stores in the city. The wards were soon filled and all patients who could be moved were taken from their beds

to make room for the burned men." [25] The overflow were cared for at a temporary facility set up by Standard Steel at the Diamond Skating Rink, in back of the YMCA. Twelve men who were not severely burned were taken there, and several physicians cared for them, the rest of the doctors working with the injured at the BCGH.

The newspaper praised the Butler Hospital superintendent and nurses:

The manner in which Mrs. Reinhart, hospital superintendent, and assistants performed their duties under the terrible stress reflected great credit upon their managerial ability. With every ward in the hospital filled, to have half a hundred men rushed into the hospital within an hour was an unlooked-for contingency. But the nurses were equal to the task. They at once placed cots and blankets at the disposal of the men who brought the injured into the building. Chairs were placed in the hallway. On these the men who were not so seriously injured were seated until cots could be gotten and places fixed in the reception room and the offices. [26]

The company was so grateful for the hospital's prompt and capable response that one year later they gave the hospital a check for $5,000.

More Growth

Once again the hospital needed to grow, and in 1907 the state legislature appropriated $10,000 for building purposes, which helped to finance the South Wing, increasing the capacity to sixty beds. The legislature also appropriated $10,000 for maintenance during the two succeeding years.

However, the mainstay of the hospital was still its Ladies' Association, whose members worked to purchase supplies for the new rooms and sewed endlessly. They organized a donation day that brought many contributions and a "cushion social" that provided fifty cushions, thirteen hassocks, and three rocking chairs.

Such donations and contributions were the lifeblood of the hospital. The report for the quarter ending May 31, 1907 lists 1,372 patients treated entirely free, 40 patients paying less than $7 per week; 257 paying $7 per week; 161 paying more than $7, but less than $12; and 438 paying more than $12.

Meanwhile, the hospital also reported that the training school for nurses had nineteen graduates, eleven in training, seven girls in uniform, four on probation, and five applicants.

The Industrial Club and Public Health

The influx of immigrant families to Lyndora had not gone unnoticed by the ladies of the town. Concerned for these new arrivals—especially the children—sixty women of the community, led by Margaret Brandon, formed the Industrial Club of Butler in 1902, another major volunteer effort. These women gave their time to teach kindergarten classes for the children and sewing classes for their mothers. Mrs. DeWitt Breaden, last president of the organization, wrote in a letter: "As many as ten or fifteen ladies of the town would go down to Lyndora to the hall that was used to conduct classes. . . . We were allowed the use of the building and, from our membership dues, we bought the material to sew with."

Eventually the members felt the need for a trained social worker/nurse who could go into the homes to teach sanitation and better living practices to the mothers, as well as cooking and sewing. They hired Anna Brown, a registered nurse who had trained at the Irene Kauffman House in Pittsburgh. She began work on June 1, 1911, and held the position for twenty-six years, an experience she later recalled with great pleasure. She was employed by the club with financial assistance from a number of churches, as well as from the Standard Steel Car Company.

Years later, Brown recounted her time when she was the first (and only) "health nurse" in the district. She began by going house to house, to explain that she would provide baby care and bedside nursing when anyone was ill. Once established, she taught the principles of sanitation, the importance of screens and proper disposal of garbage. The infant mortality rate in the area was "appallingly high," so Brown taught the mothers how to sterilize bottles, nipples, and milk. That first year there was a significant drop in the infant mortality rate.

Brown wrote:

Our first responsibility was to minister to the sick, and to those made needy by a death in the family, illness, or unemployment, and to help them until they could help themselves. . . . However, our ultimate aim was a healthy mind in a healthy body, and while we . . . maintained our nursing service for all, we expanded to include other worthwhile activities. Our reward has been to see the numberless boys and girls who grew up in the community go out into the world to take their places as doctors, nurses, teachers, businessmen, and skilled workers.

A newspaper account of July 11, 1911, shows the work accomplished by Anna Brown during the first ten days of July:

No. of patients visited 24
No. of visits made 54
No. of office patients 12
No. of patients bathed 17
No. of clinic patients bathed 17
Money collected $40
Modified milk and prepared barley water and rice water were given to several babies at clinics.
Patients have been prescribed for by their family physician and where they have none their parents were directed to secure physicians.

The total amount of money expended is $75, and the present balance is $95.15 [27]

One of the "worthwhile activities" Brown added was to help supply the children with books. Clare McJunkin, the librarian of the Butler Public Library, installed a circulating library in Brown's office. One day each week McJunkin distributed the books and held a story hour for the children. Brown said, "They read the books avidly, and then told the stories to their fathers and mothers, thus helping along the process of Americanization."

Brown added:

Volunteer work in the settlement was undertaken by some of the Butler churches. Four or five women from a church came down one evening a week to Lyndora and taught sewing to those eager to learn. It was indeed a difficult task to teach the intricacies of pattern fitting and cutting to those who spoke no English, and it is a tribute to the volunteers that they succeeded admirably.

The nursing and social work were all in a day's work to those of us trained in the profession, but it took vision and courage for the Industrial Club to undertake the project with the help of the Standard Steel Car Company. My own personal reward has been in doing a job that I loved.

According to one Lyndora resident, " My childish opinion of Brown was that she was like an angel. She just seemed to come flying in whenever we had trouble. The worse the trouble, the quicker she seemed to come."

Brown was indeed known as "the angel of Lyndora."

World War I and the Flu Epidemic

World War I

he first World War began in Europe in 1914. In April of 1917, following accelerated submarine attacks against all shipping headed for Britain, the United States also declared war on Germany.

Dr. Robert Greer, the prominent local surgeon who had organized the relief effort in the typhoid epidemic, was now the moving spirit behind the creation and management of a local chapter of the Red Cross and served as its first president—a post he was to hold for the next twenty-nine years.

Three months after its organization, the local chapter initiated a fund drive for $60,000 for war relief. By the twenty-fifth of the month the newspaper reported that the chapter would exceed its goal, raising as much as $100,000. Throughout the rest of the war the chapter organized groups to knit gloves and make tunics for the soldiers overseas.

Between 1917 and 1918, 3,000 Red Cross chapters were formed nationwide to help with the war effort. The organization initially concentrated on fund-raising, but soon expanded into all kinds of disaster assistance and relief, as well as providing consistent support for veterans and their families and men and women in active service. Today the Red Cross coordinates first aid, holds CPR and water safety training classes, and recruits blood donors. The "Gray Ladies," so called because of the color of their volunteer smocks, have given hours of service at the Veterans Hospital and Butler Memorial Hospital.

Dr. Greer, who organized the Butler chapter, was a prominent surgeon and a prototypical Butler volunteer. He was a graduate of Penn State University and the University of Pennsylvania Medical School, and served an internship at Bellevue Hospital in New York before returning to Butler to practice. Mrs. Greer assisted him in his office and, although she had no formal medical training, her gentleness made her most patients' choice for removing dressings and sutures. Her grandsons remember being told that many patients would hide until Dr. Greer left to be sure that Mrs. Greer would take care of them.

Dr. Greer's practice spanned forty-six years. During that period, he served two separate terms as president of the Butler County Medical Society, and was for many years chairman of the surgical staff of Butler Hospital. His father, Judge John M. Greer, had granted the original charter for the hospital.

Greer's specialty was surgery. Edwin Howard remembers that a nurse told him that in the first hospital building Dr. Greer operated in his bare feet. Howard speculated that it was because the floor of that early operating room was terrazzo, a composite substance that conducts electricity in much the same way as carpeting. Obviously a spark of any kind could be lethal in an operating room, where such volatile anesthetics as ether and chloroform were used. Dr. Greer's solution was both practical and creative.

The Influenza Crisis

The next major crisis for both Butler Memorial Hospital and the community was the flu epidemic of 1918. The February 23 issue of *Time* magazine called this a pandemic, which killed more people in this country than all the wars put together. It seems to have started with a few cases at an army base in Kansas, but within four months it had traversed the globe, sickening millions, but killing few. Then, in August, the virus mutated into something deadly. Outbreaks of the new flu exploded throughout the world and suddenly people were dying with blood-choked lungs; they literally drowned in their own blood. From September 1918 through March 1919, it killed more than 1 percent of the people in New York City alone — 33,387 deaths! Unlike most viruses that attack the weak and the elderly, this seemed to strike hardest at the young and healthy, ages 25-34. [28]

August of 1918 was a relatively quiet month in Butler. Everyone was focused on the war in Europe, where the enemy line was now only fifty miles from Paris. There was a national appeal for 25,000 young women to join the U.S. Student Reserve and be ready to train as nurses. (At least nine Butler nurses served with either the Red Cross or the U.S. Army, a number

of them overseas.) Anna Brown announced that sanitary conditions were much improved, owing to the prosperity enjoyed by those who found steady work because of war production. Fewer children and infants were sick than during the previous year.

There were light-hearted distractions as well. Charlie Chaplin starred in a "comedy that will make you forget that there is no ice in the refrigerator at home." It was titled *The Flirt*, and was declared "a scream from start to finish." [29]

On September 23, a brief note in *The Daily Citizen* mentioned that there were 5,324 cases of "Spanish" influenza in the army camps. By October 2, at a meeting of the Butler City Council, a letter from the state board of health asked the local board to report all cases of flu and see that they were quarantined.

Just two days later, the Pennsylvania Commissioner of Health ordered that every place of public amusement and saloon in the state be closed because of the flu epidemic. The newspaper commented, "This is the most sweeping closing order ever issued by the public board of health." The paper estimated that there were about five hundred cases in the city of Butler, but the figures could not be confirmed because, since flu had not been classified as a contagious disease, doctors had not been obliged to report them before. Furthermore, the symptoms often varied, and some cases were inevitably misdiagnosed. [30]

On October 5, the state board of health announced that all churches, schools, saloons, lodges, and, in fact, all places of assembly were to be closed indefinitely. Proprietors of large stores were asked to allow no unnecessary crowding.

The next day, when Dr. E.T. Maxwell addressed the Butler City Council, he told them, "Influenza is the most contagious of all diseases. It is known that in an epidemic 30 to 50 percent of a city are affected. . . . From 2 to 10 percent of these go into an acute

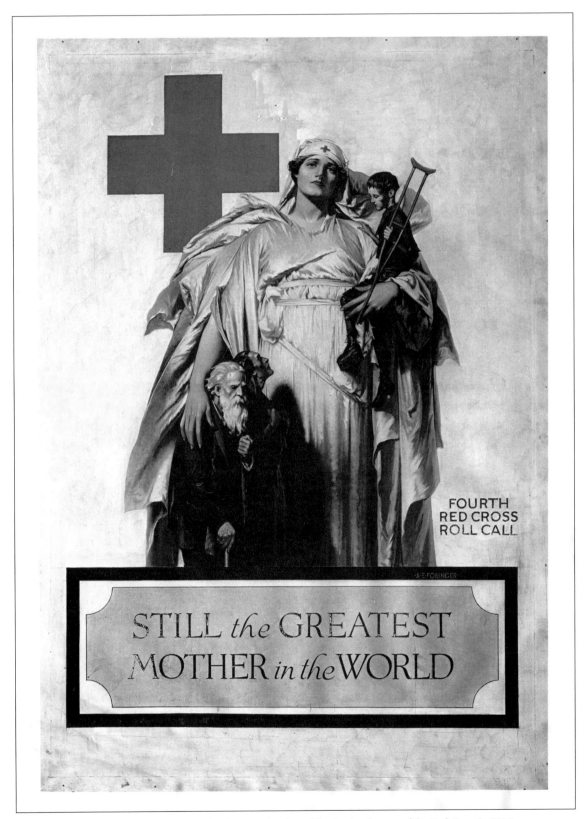

FOURTH
RED CROSS
ROLL CALL

STILL *the* GREATEST
MOTHER *in the* WORLD

The U.S. entry into the war provided the impetus for the organization of the Butler chapter of the Red Cross in 1918. Courtesy of the Red Cross stage of pneumonia. From those who are thrown into this stage 50 to 75 percent die."

He went on to say, "There are not sufficient nurses or physicians to cope with the disease. Six nurses are down at the present time. . . . The draft and the war have depleted all our ranks." *The Butler Eagle* reported, "Probably never before has Butler been so unprepared to meet such a crisis . . . . Eight doctors are in the service, one is ready to leave and one is sick." [31]

By the middle of the month there were more than 2,000 cases in Butler City alone; three nurses were sent from Harrisburg to help as visiting nurses. Dr. Greer, as president of the Red Cross, called for volunteers and pledged the support of the local chapter with nursing and supplies.

The epidemic hit Lyndora hard. Brown recalled:

We worked day and night caring for those stricken, but it was humanly impossible to care for all the rapidly mounting cases. . . . It was truly heartbreaking each morning to note by the crepe and the flowers on the doors how many of our friends had slipped away in the night. I especially remember the birth of a baby girl two hours before her mother died of flu. The father, with an already large family, could not care for the tiny one, so we obtained a desirable home for her through the Children's Aid Society, and she was adopted.

From an article by Kelly Garrett in the October 18, 1998, Butler Eagle:

Funeral homes ran out of caskets early in October. There are accounts of burials being delayed as long as ten days while caskets were sent from the other parts of the state—parts that were also fighting the same deadly disease. George Kmetz, 81, who now lives in Harmony, said his mother told him about his uncle dying from the flu on Halloween night, 1918.

"They had to wait to get a casket for three or four days, and meanwhile his infant son was sick," Kmetz said. "His son died two days after my uncle and they buried them together in the same casket five days after the son died."

There are also reports of mass graves in several cemeteries. [32]

On November 5, *The Butler Eagle* announced that the worst of the epidemic was past; there had been only four deaths the preceding twenty-four hours, as opposed to fifteen during the same time period the week before.

With the worst seemingly over, schools and theaters reopened and the restrictions on funerals due to coffin delivery were lifted. Although there were continuing deaths from pneumonia and outbreaks here and there through 1920, the virus had apparently lost its strength. The total for the city alone, according to *The Butler Eagle* on November 15, was 7,877 cases, with 260 deaths from flu from October 1 to November 15, 1918.

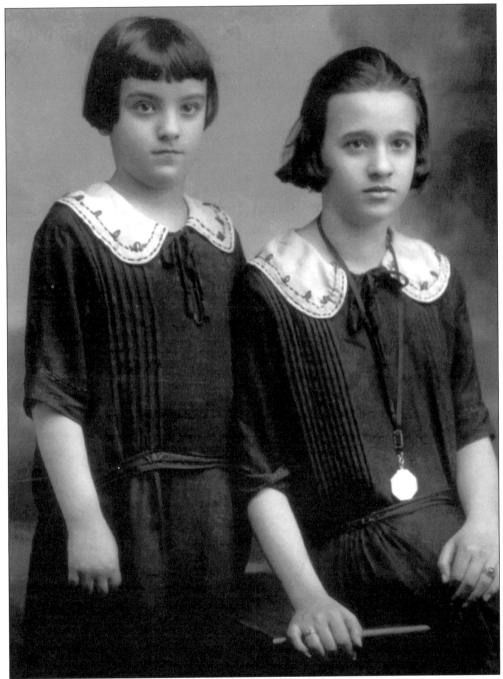

Josephine Ripper and her sister as children. She remembers: I lived in Evans City. There were eight children in the family and our whole family had influenza. My father was a shoemaker and had a grocery store and a fruit store. My brother Anthony and I were so sick no one expected us to live, but we did. My mother (she was 34 - she got married at 15) and her 16-year-old sister both died. There were funeral wreaths on every door, but the rest of us survived. The youngest child was only six months old. My father's friends helped with the children, especially the baby—he always brought her home in the evening. He raised all of us—he did a wonderful job. Courtesy of Josephine Ripper

On January 28, the Butler Memorial Hospital president in his year-end report announced that during the flu epidemic the sickness of the nurses "almost resulted in closing the hospital at a time when its services were badly needed." Five hospital employees died, four nurses and a cook. He also announced that the hospital was free from debt ... and that the average cost per patient was less than most.

He went on to make a case for a whole new hospital building, since the present building was too small and there was no way to build another addition.

It would be five years before that came to pass.

Memories Of The Flu Epidemic

Alice Fair: I was 12 years old and I lived on a farm in Washington Township; my father drove the hearse for undertakers in North Washington and Bruin. I remember him going out very early in the morning for funerals—so many, many times. My mother's sister died of the flu. In Mount Vernon cemetery off Route 38 there is one part that has no gravestones—that was because in the little mining communities around so many people were dying, a lot of them foreigners with no relatives and not much money. They had to be buried and that's where they are.

Helen Pride Wimer: I was eight years old. I remember everything was closed, schools and all. Two nights I hemorrhaged, my pillow was soaked with blood. My sister Mary was delirious. I remember some time earlier I had been to a wedding in the Catholic Church that was so romantic. Later, the bride died of flu after her baby was born. Another woman we knew died and left six children.

Jean Pfabe: We lived on Franklin Street. I remember they blocked the street with yellow ribbon when someone got sick, so that the ice wagon and other vehicles wouldn't make a lot of noise and bother the sick people. I remember I couldn't understand why so many people were dying. My mother got herbs from the drugstore, and cooked them with onion and put them in little bags we wore around our necks. We hated them, but none of the kids who wore them got the flu. (The herb was evil-smelling asafetida, which may well have kept everyone at a safe distance.)

Margaret Traggai of Cabot remembered her relatives talking about a cemetery near West Winfield. Bodies were piled on carts and taken to the cemetery where several were buried in each grave—some merely wrapped in sheets, without coffins.*

*Goldinger, Ralph and Fetters, Audrey, Butler, The Second Hundred Years

The Twenties

Rotary's Crippled Children's Clinic

n Butler County, those who volunteer are never idle. The Butler Rotary Club started the Butler County Society for Crippled Children in 1922.

The Butler County Society for Crippled Children was part of the national organization (later known as the Easter Seal Society for Crippled Children and later still, just the Easter Seal Society). In 1994, the Butler chapter disaffiliated from the national organization, becoming a local independent agency now known as Lifesteps. The mission has broadened considerably since those early days. The agency now offers a network of services for those special needs, including a pre-school and a child care program, free developmental screenings, a Family Care Mobile Library, and a Geriatric Adult Day Health Services program for the chronically ill and disabled elderly. A program of evening child care provides care for children of working parents, especially single mothers. Lifesteps also provides day programs and community homes for adults with mental retardation. But in the 1920s, the society's primary function was to run a clinic for crippled children.

1920s Medicines

LeRoy Kuhn remembers the purveyors of snake oil and miracles in the 1920s by travelling "medicine men." A standard part of "medical delivery" in the 1920s was the hawking of "wonder remedies" by travelling "medicine men:"

"A hot summer in a small town was a pretty dull place for a growing boy. But for one week it was exciting, more fun than taking the train trip to Butler. The medicine man had come to town. A man and a woman with their teenage kid and a helper. . . set up on a vacant lot and were ready for six nights.

"From their shaky stage they put on short plays with lots of fun and laughter. They told funny jokes using names of local people. When the crowd seemed jovial and excited the medicine man came on the stage to sell the most wonderful remedy in the world for every ache and pain. Dressed in his flowing garments he told of the thousands of people he had restored to good health. When the people seemed excited and happy he came off the stage and started to sell this marvelous cure-all for one dollar a bottle. For every sale you put in a vote for the prettiest girl in town. Hen Thompson was circulating in the crowd getting votes for his daughter. My dad wasn't going to let that happen, he laid down two ten-dollar bills and voted twenty times for his Sarah. The medicine did contain a cathartic and was mostly alcohol so it did make people feel good for a time."

Other medicines were sold over the counter in places like Kuhn's Country Store. One example was Kuhn Saval, a jar of cream that could heal a cut or bruise in a very short time. Orders came in from all over the country. But the inventor, who made it all himself and delivered it in a little old Ford, refused to expand his business. When the government required him to list all the ingredients, he stopped making it.

Another wonderful remedy was Asiatic Balsam, made in Parker by a Mr. Turk. It was developed for men who got burned in the oil fields. A bad burn would heal, or at least improve, almost the next day, according to Kuhn. After Turk died, the family tried to make the balm, but it wasn't the same; it made burns worse. [33]

The Butler County Medical Society and Auxiliary

In 1923, the Butler County Medical Society had a membership of fifty-four doctors. Their monthly meetings focused on medical problems of general interest at the time: goiter, especially in the young; syphilis (the U.S. Public Health Service recommended treatment for three years for the average case and observation for five years "before marriage should be considered"); pneumonia (light diet, fresh air—not too much or too cold—and hydrotherapy).

The long-term effects of radiation were just beginning to be understood. A doctor from Kane spoke on the subject of cancer and its treatment. He recommended x-ray and radium treatments, found to be effective, he said, in large cancers but not small ones. He went on to say, "Radiation seems to have a deleterious effect on those handling it and therefore is not absolutely harmless to patients, and may even cause death if used in large doses." Protective shielding was yet to come.

The society was also concerned about blocking a pardon for Dr. Kartub. According to medical society records, in 1917, Dr. Kartub, working with a justice of the peace and another man who posed as the beneficiary, concocted a murderous insurance scam. First they insured a very sick man, then the doctor fed him a lethal dose of chloral hydrate. The trio then collected the insurance. At the trial, Dr. Kartub confessed to a similar murder the year before.

The society went on record as absolutely opposed to any pardon for the criminally enterprising physician.

In 1924, there was a statewide move to form a medical auxiliary of doctors' wives. Dr. Mary Brook St. Clair of the Butler County Medical Society and wife of Dr. H.B. St. Clair, organized the Woman's Medical Auxiliary for the State of Pennsylvania the following year, and Mrs. Robert Greer of Butler served as the first president. In later years, the auxiliary, which met once a month, established a scholarship fund for nurses, which they supported with many fund-raising projects.

The New Hospital

The movement for a new hospital, which was begun before World War I, was gaining ground. By 1920 the hospital's board of directors and the Chamber of Commerce had established a committee to raise half a million dollars for a new building. The board of trustees bought ten acres on the summit of a hill within city limits, on the White estate. It was no longer simple to build a hospital; all plans had to be approved by the state Departments of Public Welfare, Labor and Industry, and the Arts Commission. Once the plans were approved, the committee started a second campaign in 1924 that raised a quarter of a million dollars more.

The board decided that this new building would be called Butler County Memorial Hospital, in memory of all who served in World War I. They obtained a new charter on November 25, 1924, which stated that the object was "the maintenance of a hospital as a public charity and a training school for nurses, as a memorial to all of the soldiers and sailors from Butler County who served the United States or its allies in the World War, and the Hospital shall be known as Butler County Memorial Hospital."

Six days later the old hospital was closed and the patients moved to the new facility on East Brady Street. During its first twenty-seven years of operation, the old Butler County General Hospital had received 22,930 patients; 10,419 surgical operations had been performed; and 1,209 babies had been born there.

The first patient admitted to the new building was George Martin, who was "painfully but not seriously injured by an explosion in the pipe fitting department of the Standard Steel Car Company."

Here is a description of the new building from *The Butler Eagle:*

There are four wards on the first floor and six on the second floor besides about fifty private rooms. The third floor is being used for nurses' quarters. On the fourth floor there is a finely equipped operating room, well lighted and spotlessly clean. There are also special operating rooms on the first and

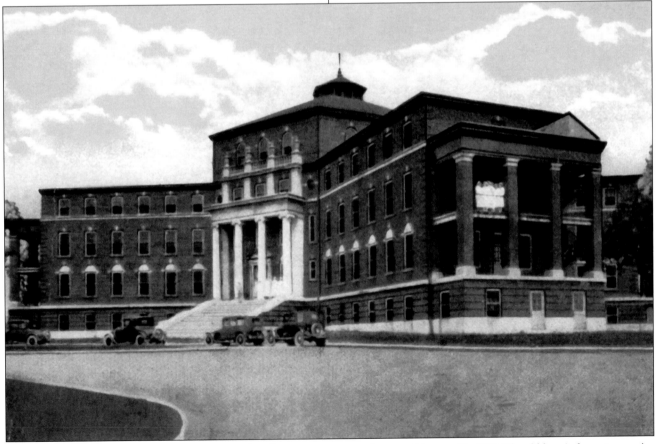

The new Butler County Memorial Hospital was officially open to accept patients on February 18, 1925. The old hospital was to remain open until all patients could be safely transported to the new facility. Courtesy of Butler Memorial Hospital

second floors. . . . A complete system of lights instead of bells is used to call nurses into private rooms.

The institution is one of the finest in the state and is expected to handle any emergency that may arise. [34]

The new building was called the "X building" because of its shape. Mae Vensel, a nurse at the hospital, remembered that the day after the move the staff had to perform both an emergency appendectomy and a mastoid operation.

The average daily census for the first year in the new building was forty-one. There were twenty-five students in the nursing school; by the next year there were thirty.

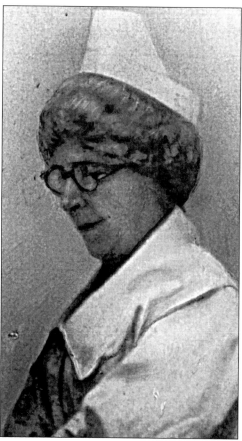

Miss Rose Whitney was to continue as hospital superintendent with Miss Mabel Campbell as her assistant. Courtesy of Butler Memorial Hospital Nurses' Alumnae Association

The new hospital had its opportunity to handle a major accident. In 1927, a truck carrying 440 quarts of nitroglycerine overturned on Lick Hill, northeast of Butler, on the Chicora Road. The resulting explosion blew the driver and his companion literally to pieces. According to *The Butler Eagle*, the blast shook every building in the city of Butler and its effects were felt for miles. The explosion ripped a great hole in the road and the telephone and telegraph wires were downed. Seven people were admitted to the hospital, 75 people were homeless and were temporarily housed in the old East Butler Hotel, which was hastily refitted with cots and donated necessities. [35]

The Salvation Army and the Red Cross came to the rescue— the latter established a relief center for donations, and, together with *The Butler Eagle*, raised $4,000. Once again, the hospital and the community's volunteers had dealt with a crisis with dispatch and efficiency.

In 1928, Mabel Campbell was named hospital superintendent, to succeed Rose Whitney, who had died. Everything seemed to be going well for the hospital, for Butler, for the country.

Then, in 1929, the stock market crashed, triggering the Great Depression. Its consequences were not immediately realized. Indeed, owing to its economic diversity, Butler did not feel the effects as soon or as severely as many other parts of the country.

But the worst was yet to come.

Meanwhile, the Ladies' Hospital Association, which had disbanded with the closing of the old hospital, reorganized as the Auxiliary to the Butler County Memorial Hospital. By July 1926, the organization had 127 paid members. Once again, the women were making the necessary sheets, pillow cases, and towels and raising cash in a variety of creative ways. They set aside $1,000 to beautify the grounds and planted 2,100 trees and shrubs. From 1927 to 1932 the auxiliary held a series of benefits, parties, teas, and plays to raise money, all of which went to support the hospital's mission.

The Depression Years

The Great Depression

y 1931, banks across the country had failed and there was massive unemployment everywhere, including Butler. In April of 1932, a relief committee initiated a house-to-house canvass to raise funds for needy families. The Red Cross distributed free flour, and the Butler Township school board announced that they would accept contributions for a milk fund for undernourished children.

Butler Hospital also felt the effects of the Great Depression. In May, a headline in *The Butler Eagle* announced that the hospital was "Low on Finances, May Close Doors." The problem was an ongoing deficit of $2,000 a month. The cause: first, more charity patients; and, second, the appropriation from the state did not cover the cost of operating the hospital—$3.00 per day per patient. This happened because the total reimbursement from the state was based on the previous number of free patients instead of the actual number, which had increased tremendously.

In May, the board of directors announced a campaign to raise $25,000 to cover the deficit. They met with service clubs and civic groups to explain the need. A committee from the medical society visited other comparable hospitals to compare cost, efficiency, and service, and returned with the information that Butler compared favorably in every respect. Other hospitals were reporting similar problems. The Oil City Hospital's monthly deficit was $3,000 per month, in spite of an endowment and help from the Oil City Community Chest. New Castle's Jameson Hospital was also reporting financial difficulties.

By the middle of June, the campaign had topped its $25,000 goal, with the doctors contributing $4,000. Once again, the community had rallied to support Butler Hospital and its mission.

In 1932, Mabel Campbell resigned as superintendent and was replaced by Mabel Grace Wilson. Managing a hospital was becoming more complex.

Sarver Hall

Maintaining the nurses training school continued to be a major priority for the hospital and its board. From 1925 to 1927, nursing students had been housed on the third floor of the hospital, but when it became necessary to take over the space for patient care, the nurses were moved to the old hospital building.

In 1938, however, A.H. Sarver, a former Butler resident and an executive with General Motors, offered

Medical Memories –
"Every illness meant a housecall"

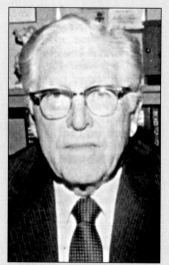

Dr. Coulter began his practice in 1935 and retired in 1992, but continued to take care of his "old ladies"—mostly, he said, a matter of stopping in to see them and listen to their complaints. But the cost of medical malpractice made even that impractical.

Courtesy of Butler Memorial Hospital

Dr. Clinton Coulter began practicing medicine in Parker City in 1935 as a newly licensed physician. His family doctor in Wesley, southern Venango County, had suggested Parker, since the doctor there was approaching retirement. His father and brother said the place was "in terrible shape but a good place to start."

Dr. Coulter recalled that when he drove over to check it out he passed the old town doctor on the street:

He took me in to his dusty, grimy old office, handed me the keys and said I was the new doc. He said I could rent the equipment and his office and use up his supplies for $20 a month. I had $30 to my name. So I scrubbed the place from top to bottom and slept in the back room until I got married. I stayed in that office until 1953.

In those days, for a country doctor every illness meant a house call. It took a lot of time to drive around on those mud roads. I always figured I'd had a good day if I saw five patients, because I had to drive all over the countryside to see them. So you surely didn't get rich quick.

Practicing medicine was very different. There were no antibiotics. The practice of medicine had not changed much from 1900 to World War II. The same drugs were available: morphine, aspirin, quinine and an array of laxatives. If a patient contracted pneumonia there was nothing to treat it with. You accepted a 40 percent mortality rate among your pneumonia patients. Many diseases have all but been eradicated since World War II. I haven't seen a case of typhoid fever since before the war.

the board of directors a gift of $170,000 for a nurses' residence, provided it was a memorial to his wife, Ottie Pillow Sarver, and daughter, Eleanor Sarver Allen. Immediately, the board began making plans to build Sarver Hall.

Tuberculosis and Deshon Hospital

Tuberculosis (TB), sometimes called "the white plague" or "consumption," is an ancient disease, contagious and potentially fatal. Its symptoms include a chronic cough and "night sweats." Patients wake in the night drenched with a cold sweat and short of breath. Today's antibiotics can usually cure even the most advanced cases of tuberculosis, though the patient must continue treatment long after he feels completely well so that all the slow-growing bacteria are killed. But in the 30s, TB, which had a high mortality rate, was often a long drawn-out disease, taking its toll on families as well as patients.

The January, 1930 meeting of the Butler County Medical Society focused on "Tuberculosis, Its Care in Butler County." Dr. R.M. Christie, the retiring president, recapped the history of the state

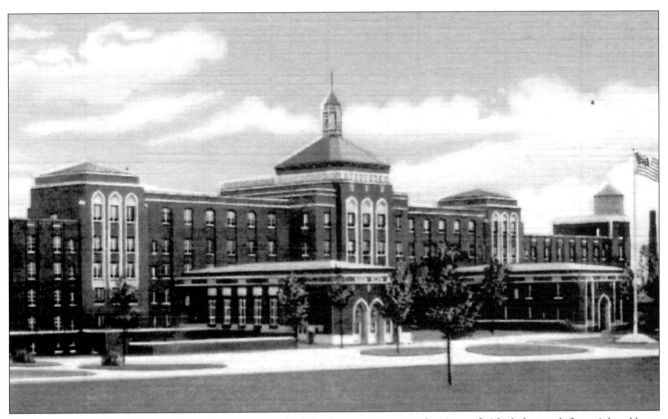

The Western Pennsylvania Tuberculosis Sanatorium was built by the state in 1939. When it was finished, the state's financial problems were such that no patients were admitted, and it remained empty until World War II when it was acquired by the United States Army Medical Department. Today it is the Veterans Administration Medical Center. Courtesy of Susan Vieira-Kane

tuberculosis clinic in Butler County, which had been established in 1907. He explained that there were 128 such clinics in Pennsylvania, which served as clearing houses for tuberculosis patients. Nevertheless, he pointed out that "the state sanatoriums cannot take care of all the tuberculosis cases, and do not wish to take advanced cases. Butler County has no place to send advanced cases and there are at least twelve such cases in the county receiving very meager care." He went on to say that the county commissioners had discussed establishing such a facility, possibly together with an adjoining county, and he suggested the county society pass a resolution in support of the project. This project did not gain momentum until 1939, when a sanatorium was built by the state on New Castle Road.

In October 1942, the United States Army Medical

Department renamed the sanatorium Deshon General Hospital and reopened it as a general medical and surgical facility, with a special center for hearing disability. Throughout the war, patients were sent to Deshon to recover from their war-related injuries. With characteristic hospitality, members of the Butler community opened their homes to the families of these patients, providing them with a place to stay when they came to visit. In 1946, after the war, the Department of Veterans Affairs took control of the hospital to care for World War II veterans and today this hospital is named the Department of Veterans Affairs Medical Center.

Originally, there were five hundred beds in the medical center for general medical/surgical patients and five hundred for tuberculosis patients, but in 1951 it became a specialty hospital devoted to tuberculosis.

The facility underwent another change in 1959 when it became apparent that TB had become treatable with some of the new antibiotics. In 1963, the hospital was authorized to admit all general and surgical patients. With health care reform during the 1980s and 1990s, the VA Medical Center has evolved into a primary medical care facility offering outpatient care and acute inpatient care as well as a comprehensive continuum of extended, transitional and mental health services.

World War II and After

The years during World War II were difficult; not only did the hospital lose physicians and nurses to the war effort, but support and maintenance staff as well.

Once more the volunteers of the community pitched in to help. The Red Cross trained local women as nurses' aides. These volunteers worked many hours, staying with post-operative patients and helping in any way they could. The Women's Auxiliary fixed lunches and dinners for the doctors, and members of the medical auxiliary helped in the kitchen as well.

Following the war, in 1945, the Women's Auxiliary of Butler County Memorial Hospital was reorganized under the leadership of Louise Hetrick, who had worked as a volunteer aide during the war. Their first major project was a self-sustaining snack bar to serve doctors, nurses, and patients' families. The board of directors loaned the auxiliary $2,500 to remodel a small room on the main floor and purchase equipment. Six months later, in July of 1946, the Hostess Shoppe and Travel Cart were a reality: including a snack bar, a counter for three customers, magazines,

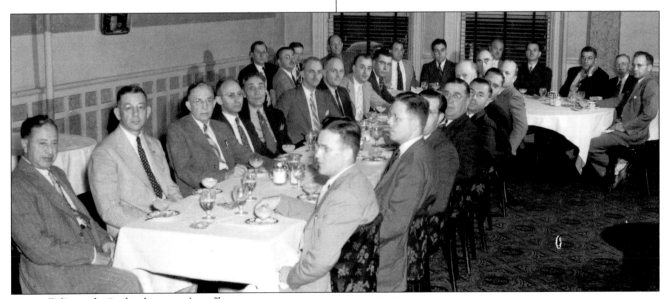

Farewell dinner for Butler doctors going off to war.   Courtesy of Butler County Medical Society

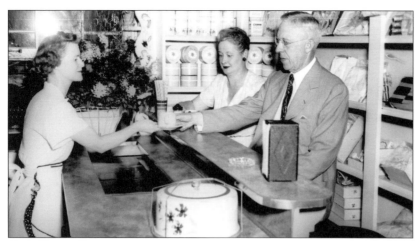

Early Hostess Shoppe   Courtesy of Butler Memorial Hospital Auxiliary

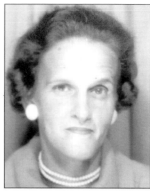

Louise Hetrick, one of the founders of the Hostess Shoppe and an Auxilian who also helped to regenerate the hospital Auxiliary.

Courtesy of Butler Memorial Hospital Auxiliary

and small gifts. Katherine Davy was the first paid director, but auxiliary members staffed the shoppe. They repaid the loan within a year.

A year later the shoppe had to be enlarged, and in 1948 when the hospital expansion was discussed, the auxiliary pledged $10,000 toward the cost of a new shoppe in the new wing—one of the largest donations to the building fund.

World War II ended in 1945, but the war had changed the practice of medicine forever. Medicines and techniques developed to treat soldiers would now benefit civilians. The development of penicillin and other antibiotics meant that doctors could cure a whole host of formerly untreatable diseases. Physicians no longer expected 40 percent of their pneumonia patients to die; most survived. And along with these wonderful new drugs came a change in patients' attitudes. As Dr. Coulter said, "They now expected to be cured." Furthermore, from now on, medical technology would increase exponentially, adding immeasurably to the ability to cure or prolong life.

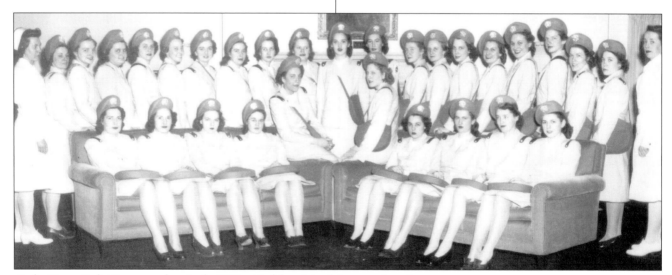

Butler Nurse Cadet Corp. members in the 1940s; 46 of these joined the armed services.   Courtesy of Butler Memorial Hospital Nurses' Alumnae Association

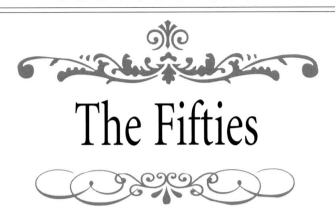

The Fifties

Medicine in the Fifties

edical treatment before the 1950s was almost like another world. Doctors kept patients who had cataract surgery in bed and did not allow them to move their heads for a week; they often placed sandbags on each side to keep the head still. Now this surgery is accomplished with lasers, in the doctor's office, and the patient goes home immediately afterward.

In the forties, women stayed in the hospital for ten days to two weeks after childbirth. In the fifties, they usually stayed for a week, sometimes less with no complications. Now, with no complications, mothers go home in about forty-eight hours.

Gall bladder surgery was a major operation with a large incision, and patients were kept in bed a week to ten days before they were allowed to walk. Now it is almost microsurgery and patients are up and moving almost immediately.

Heart attack patients were kept in bed two weeks and not permitted to move, which increased the possibility of complications. Now doctors have much better results by getting patients up and moving as soon as possible, even after bypass surgery. Much more is known now about the therapeutic value of exercise and special diets.

Dr. Ernie Moore began to practice in Butler in 1950, when doctors still made house calls and carried the "little black bag." "Trouble was finding space for so many medications for home treatment. And house calls took so much time. Many medical problems that today would be treated in the hospital were treated at home."

Dr. Ralph Weaver, former head of the pathology department at BMH, came to Butler in 1952. He recalled that at that time there were few specialists; many of the general practitioners (today's family practice specialists) did general surgery and obstetrics. In the fifties, medicine became much more specialized, and eventually family practice was recognized as a specialty.

Polio and the March of Dimes

Many older residents remember that, along with vacations, summertime brought the threat of infantile paralysis (poliomyelitis). The country's attention first focused on polio during the presidency of Franklin D. Roosevelt, its most famous victim. In 1938, the National Foundation for Infantile Paralysis was organized in New York for the purpose of finding a cause, prevention, and cure for the disease, as well as providing proper care for polio victims. Chapters were organized in every county in the United States. The Butler chapter was organized in March of 1941, with Dr. John Burn, pediatrician, as its first president, and immediately went to work to raise money. That first year there was one case in the chapter's files. The year 1949 represented a major epidemic: 42,375 cases were reported in the nation, with 58 in Butler County. (Twenty cases per 100,000 is considered an epidemic.) By 1950, there were 113 recorded cases in Butler County.

Care for polio patients— the treatments, the lengthy and costly rehabilitation—was made possible by the yearly national fund drive in January, the March of Dimes, or Mothers' March. On a specified evening, church bells and whistles in each community signaled the start of the one-hour march, and women went door-to-door asking for contributions.

Mary Hulton Phillips (far right), who organized Butler's first March of Dimes—the second March in the country. It was so efficiently organized by Mary Phillips and her committee that the national organization borrowed Butler's maps and plans for their instruction booklet for other chapters. Mrs. Phillips, who chaired the March for many years and also served at the division level, is forever identified with the Mothers' March.

Courtesy of The Butler Eagle

doses were needed to complete the immunization.) Doctors and nurses contributed their time, and the vaccine was given free to 78,000 Butler County residents. The vaccine was easy to dispense—a few drops on a sugar cube. No child objected to that!

Because polio is now largely unknown in the western hemisphere, the March of Dimes Foundation concentrates on eliminating birth defects, and they hold an annual walk-a-thon in the spring.

Firsts— the Outpatient Clinic and the Emergency Room

Meanwhile, the community was enjoying growth of both population and prosperity,

Dr. Jonas Salk developed an effective vaccine that immunized children against polio in 1955. In 1961, Dr. Albert Sabin's oral vaccine was available for distribution, and three years later the Butler County Medical Society held a countywide program to immunize all of Butler County's children. Dr. Joseph Purvis, Jr. headed the program, which took place in public school buildings throughout the county on three Sundays. (Three

with the result that Butler County Memorial Hospital again needed more beds, as well as building additions and renovations to accommodate technology.

Originally planned in 1944, a major expansion of Butler Hospital was sorely needed, but had been postponed. In 1948, Butler County Memorial Hospital initiated a building fund to expand and renovate the X Building. When completed it included: a whole new wing (the T Building), a six-story addition that opened in 1954; Nixon Hall, a sixty-four-room nurses' dormitory (in part funded by a gift from the estate of Simeon Nixon), which now accommodated 125 students; and renovation to the old facility. The new wing included an outpatient clinic. Also included was an all-new x-ray department, equipped with the latest technologies in the field.

An emergency room had been set up earlier as a one-room operation, staffed on an as-needed basis. It usually wasn't needed, since people went to their own doctors—or their doctors went to them for most treatments. In addition, many medical problems that today require hospital services, such as congestive heart failure and acute gall bladder attacks, were treated at home. The room designated was between Wards A and B on the first floor, and the equipment consisted of one cot, an oval table, a scrub sink, and two medical cupboards. A year later in 1955, however, there was room for four patients, two regular examining tables, an ear/nose/throat chair, a minor examining table, two regular

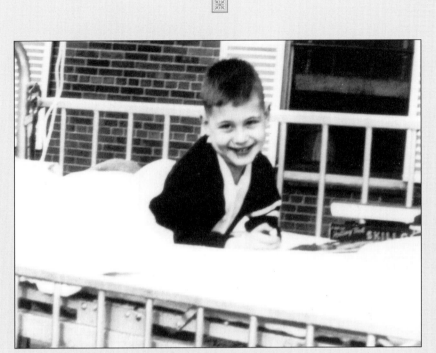

Joe Randig, Butler poster boy for the Mother's March of Dimes
Courtesy of Joe Randig and The Butler Eagle

Joe Randig, shown here as the March of Dimes Poster Boy, contracted polio in 1952, two weeks after he started first grade. His home was quarantined for two weeks—food and supplies were brought by relatives who would set the items on the porch and then step back, while someone came out to get them.

Following a stay at Municipal Hospital, Joe was admitted to the D. T. Watson Home for Crippled Children in Sewickley, to stay for the next 20 months. Initial treatment was hot packs, muscle stretching and re-education. (Those unable to breathe on their own were placed in an iron lung.) After months of physical therapy, Joe was fitted with braces on his legs, a back brace and crutches—and learned to walk all over again. All of Joe's treatment was paid for by the National Foundation.

Joe remembered that in 1960 he was going to Butler Hospital outpatient therapy department for follow-up therapy. He said, "My therapist, Al Peretic, gave me a leather wallet. Leatherworking was his hobby so he made a real nice, hand-tooled leather wallet for me. He explained that my spine was starting to curve and suggested that I sit with the wallet under my right hip. This would keep my spine straight while sitting."

sinks, one scrub sink, medical cupboards, desks, and two-bowl sinks.

In 1955, the administration added a full-time emergency room nurse, with the medical staff taking turns in the emergency room from midnight until 8:00 a.m. The nurse on call always called the family doctor first, then notified the doctor on call if there was no family doctor or if he was unavailable. By 1960, a gynecological examining table and another bed had been added, and there were five nurses on duty.

Dr. Goehring's wife remembered that the heat in the operat-

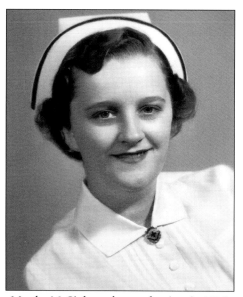

Martha McGinley at her graduation in 1954. Ms. McGinley was the first full-time nurse assigned to the Emergency Department—which meant Monday through Friday and every other weekend off. There was no regular physician assigned. Courtesy of Martha McGinley

ing rooms in those days was brutal, not only in summer but year round. It was so intense that during every operation a nurse was stationed to wipe the perspiration from the surgeon's brow. At that time, today's array of sophisticated anesthetics was not yet available. Ether was the anesthetic of choice, and a nurse administered it at the surgeon's direction, dropping it on the patients' face masks during surgery. One of the welcome improvements of the 1955 project was air conditioning added in all the operating rooms.

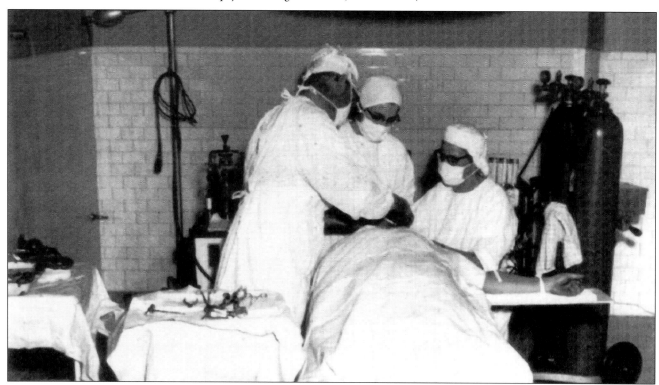

This 1940s operating room seems empty, compared with today's facility with its monitors and other high tech equipment.
Courtesy of Butler Memorial Hospital

The Sixties and Seventies

Butler County Health Department —In and Out

n the early fifties, the state legislature enacted legislation enabling second-class counties to establish county health departments. The Butler County commissioners duly established such a department in 1953, a move ratified by the voters in 1954. Butler was the first county to set up a county health department, and the county received grants from the Mellon Charitable Trust and help from advisory personnel from the University of Pittsburgh's School of Public Health.

During its brief tenure, the department ran well-baby clinics, offered visiting nurse home care, inspected restaurants, and analyzed water samples. The department also became involved in Butler County's serious water and sewage problems. Tests performed in 1959 showed that 30 percent of the public water supplies

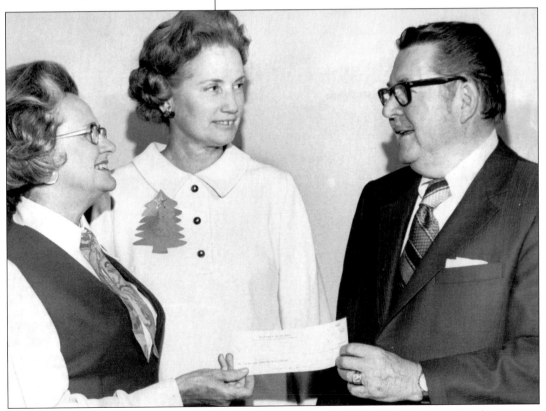

A.C. (Bert) Sewall, shown here with Auxiliary members, was named superintendent of the hospital in January 1954—the first man to assume the post. He succeeded Miss Jane Boyd. Courtesy of The Butler Eagle

and 38 percent of 508 drilled wells were unsafe. In many parts of the county, developments had permitted septic tank installations and wells on quarter-acre lots, where clay soil prevented proper absorption. The department was responsible for requiring percolation tests before a building permit could be issued in the parts of the county not served by sewers. They also established strict requirements on garbage dumps.

These stringent regulations aroused the opposition of some of the County's township supervisors, as well as those who favored development. The department's opponents were able to pass legislation to hold a referendum on whether or not to retain the department and had the ballot question phrased in such a way that to vote "yes" meant to eliminate the department. In spite of strong support from doctors and many others in the community, in November of 1960 Butler County attained the dubious distinction of being the only county in the nation to vote out a county health department.

The demise of the county health department, however, was directly responsible for the creation of the Visiting Nurses Association. The League of Women Voters had strongly supported the department, and two members of the organization, learning how important the visiting nurse home care services were to the families and physicians in the community, worked to establish a Visiting Nurses Association to provide the service. With support from the Butler County Medical Society, major employers in the county, and, finally, the Community Chest (now United Way), the VNA became a reality in 1964. The organization now provides greatly expanded services including: home health aides, hospice care, professional nursing, a variety of therapies, medical equipment and supplies, and many other services with offices that service a tri-county area.

Mental Health Focus

Although the Butler County Medical Society and the State Medical Auxiliary had cosponsored a public program on mental health in the thirties, other medical problems took precedence. It was not until the fifties that the mental health committee of the Health and Welfare Council became the first group of volunteers to concentrate on the mental health needs of Butler county. Dr. John Shadle, Butler's first psychiatrist, helped to establish a nine-bed psychiatric unit at BCMH in 1955, and that same year the Mental Health Association was born. In 1959, the Mental Health Guidance Clinic was opened following a survey of the need for such services. The need became acute in 1966, when the state hospitals returned many of their patients to the community, endorsing the concept of community care without providing adequate funding for their treatment.

Parents and community leaders concerned with a lack of programs for individuals with mental retardation and their families, organized the Association for Retarded Citizens (ARC)—Butler County in 1957. Today, among its many services, ARC—Butler County offers a variety of residential living options for adults with mental retardation; and, both sheltered and competitive employment services for people with mental retardation and other disabilities. The ARC is committed to securing for all people with mental retardation the opportunity to choose and realize their goals, of where and how they learn, live, work, and play.

Medicare and Medicaid

The social programs of the sixties included two that vitally affected both hospitals and patients. The enactment of Medicare meant a drastic change for older Americans, who typically require many medical and hospital services.

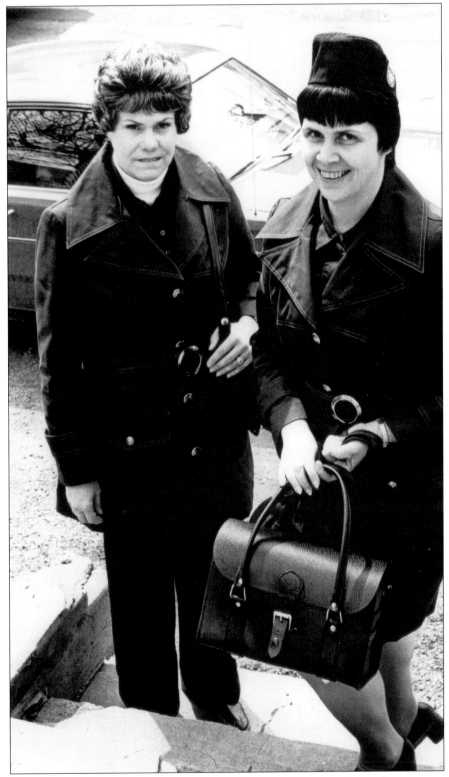

Two visiting nurses start out on their rounds in the sixties—Karen Reiser and Kim Schroerlucke. Courtesy of Visiting Nurses Association

Medical insurance, a development of the late forties and fifties, was beginning to cover more people. Medicaid, designed to pay for medical care for those who could not afford insurance, was a recognition of the free care hospitals and physicians had given for years and, in many cases, continued to give.

These developments changed the face of medical care and how it was paid for.

Because medical insurance was set up to reimburse hospital costs, not tests or outpatient treatment, patients were often admitted to the hospital for testing and sometimes minor procedures. In addition, surgical patients were typically admitted the day before surgery, and kept in the hospital for a week to ten days afterwards.

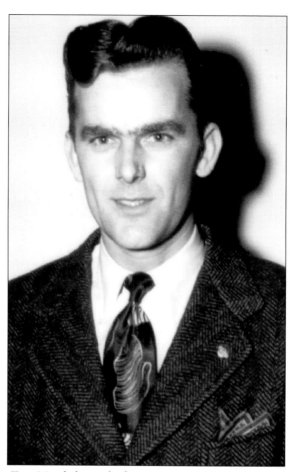

Tony Menchyk was the first patient at BMH to receive a temporary pacemaker.   Courtesy of Mrs. Tony Menchyk

wing and more beds. A new north wing, opened in 1972, increased the total number of beds to 356— the last such expansion. From then on expansions and changes were to accommodate new technology and services and to provide for the many developments in the way medical care was being delivered.

The seventies brought many more changes. In 1970, the first nuclear medicine camera arrived, and the first computer used in the finance department was a harbinger of the future. Also in 1970, the hospital added a four-bed intensive care unit. In 1971, it was expanded to ten beds, and the coronary care unit was opened. Nurse Lucille Swigart was asked to head the ICU, and

There still was not a lot to be done for heart patients, except to keep them comfortable. But by this time, more people were being admitted to the hospital because there were more options for treatment that could not be carried out at home or in the doctor's office.

The day when doctors made house calls with their little black bags was gradually disappearing.

The Seventies—and More Changes

It seemed as though every ten years Butler Memorial needed to grow and change. By 1968, Butler County Memorial Hospital was raising funds to add another

she remembered her dismay at first seeing all those monitors that no one knew how to read. That didn't last. She went to the University of Pittsburgh and learned not only to read the monitors but also the electrocardiograms. When she returned, with help from Butler cardiologists, she taught the other nurses.

Swigart also established the first cardiac crash cart that carried supplies for emergency treatment. Faye Silverio, former head nurse of the recovery room, remembered the first time they used the crash cart, on January 11, 1971. A patient came to the admissions office and sat down in the lounge. The admissions clerk could see something was wrong, so she quickly got the nursing supervisor, who called for the cart and the emergency room doctor. The patient was in cardiac arrest, but prompt treatment brought him around. He was admitted to the new ICU and made a full recovery.

According to Dr. Robert McKee, a retired BMH surgeon, the ICU is one of the most important advances in medicine. He is quick to credit the nurses for their competence, skill, and ability to evaluate patients. "They saved the day in the ICU and ER when we did not have all the medical personnel of a big city hospital," he said. The nurses, in turn, are quick to credit the doctors, who "always had time to explain and to teach." The community can be proud that BMH's ICU has consistently had a much lower than average mortality rate.

In 1972, Dr. McKee and Dr. Joseph Purvis, Jr., internist and cardiologist, installed the first temporary pacemaker in a patient. McKee had trained at the Mayo Clinic and had been involved in some of the early heart surgery there. "He wouldn't have lasted the trip to Pittsburgh without it," Dr. McKee said.

The hospital continued to make improvements in response to the needs of the times. In the seventies, they added a twenty-two-bed unit to cope with increasing alcohol abuse and drug addiction cases. The maternity unit, with rooming-in and family-centered services, reflected the changes in maternal care and delivery.

The emergency department was remodeled and enlarged, with a physician on call twenty-four hours a day. Dr. Ernie Moore has called the establishment and staffing of the emergency department the biggest improvement in today's medical scene. "Originally the doctors took turns being on call. Nowadays, with trauma such a specialty, it would never do."

By the late seventies, hospital emergency rooms were increasingly seeing patients who in previous years would have gone to a doctor's office. Many of these people believed their insurance would cover the cost of hospital emergency treatment but not treatment in a doctor's office. Increasing, too, was the number of patients with no family physician. Of necessity, the emergency department instituted triage—the practice of evaluating patients and treating the most serious cases first.

In the seventies, people also began to recognize the age-old problem of domestic abuse. In 1978, the Volunteers Against Abuse Center (VAAC) was organized, to provide help and support for women and children fleeing abusive home situations. VAAC provides safe houses for shelter and offers counseling and support to abused women, who often need help determining how to take control of their lives. Recently, VAAC and Crime Victim Services merged into one organization to better serve the people of Butler County.

Facing Difficulties

With the new wing completed, the hospital was busy and all seemed well. However, the hospital was about to enter one of its most difficult periods. The nation's economy faltered in the early seventies, and once again, the discrepancy between government reimbursement for Medicare and Medicaid, and private insurance reimbursement, and the actual costs of hospital care resulted in financial problems for BMH, as for other hospitals.

The board of directors brought in a new administrator, whose job was to manage the hospital more efficiently. Unfortunately, staffing changes, loss of important personnel, and a lack of communication between administration, board and medical staff resulted in significant deterioration of staff morale and the loss of the hospital's accreditation. The problem became so acute that the Butler Hospital Association,[36] a community group which selected the Board of Directors, voted in a new board, who in turn replaced the administrator. The new board then applied for and received accreditation. A positive result of that trying period in history was a closer working relationship between staff, administration, and the board of directors.

The last nursing class to graduate from Butler Hospital's Nurses Training Program. One of the casualties of the economic problems of the seventies was the Nursing School, which graduated its last class in 1974. During its 71 years the school graduated 1,143 nurses, and has sent its graduates to the armed forces in both wars, and on to careers in the mission field, as well as other hospitals. The school was accredited by the National League of Nursing Accreditation in 1960 and retained that distinction throughout its remaining 14 years. According to Dr. Tony Pirello, chief pathologist at the hospital for many years, many doctors were sorry to see the school close its doors, because they believed that the nurses trained in the Butler Hospital School received more hands-on training and experience than those from strictly academic programs.

Courtesy of Butler Memorial Hospital Nurses' Alumnae Association

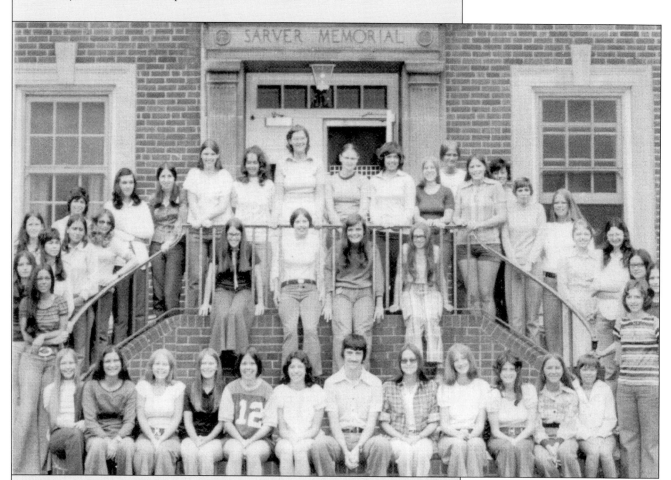

The Information Age and Community Service

The Eighties— Computers and More

 ne computer in Butler Memorial Hospital's finance department in the seventies was the forerunner of a veritable onslaught of computers in the eighties, not only in finance and administration where they provided quicker and easier registration for patients, but throughout the hospital, where they provided staff with instant access to information and patient records. Along with the computers came a flood of new technology, and the new Main Wing was constructed to accommodate it.

Spacious lab and x-ray areas were a feature of the project, as well as renovated patient areas. The accelerated growth of drug use as well as alcohol abuse (lumped together in the term "substance abuse") led to the expansion of the drug and alcohol detoxification and rehabilitation unit to 20 beds.

The outpatient department, which had originally been designated for indigent patients, had changed its role through the years and had become the primary stop for patients who needed lab work, x-ray services, or other testing that no longer included a hospital stay. In the new project, the outpatient department was enlarged and renovated to include ambulatory surgery—that is, surgery with no inpatient stay. With the improvements in technology, more and more surgical procedures could be done on an outpatient basis. Today, 70 percent of all surgery at Butler Memorial Hospital is ambulatory.

The emergency department also needed more room and more equipment: first, because of the increase in number of patients, and second, because trauma care for accident victims had become more highly specialized.

Nurse practitioner Ann McCarren, who headed the newly expanded emergency department, explained that in the past all patients from the same accident were taken to the same area, separated only by a curtain. With the new setup, patients in serious condition could be sent to either the department's specialized trauma areas or to one of twelve specialized treatment rooms. The major trauma room was equipped with heart monitors, cardiac arrest devices, and oxygen. Monitored beds in the treatment rooms were equipped with advanced cardiac life support systems.

Another improvement was the establishment of a minor care area where minor injuries, such as cuts or fractures, could receive treatment promptly without a long wait.

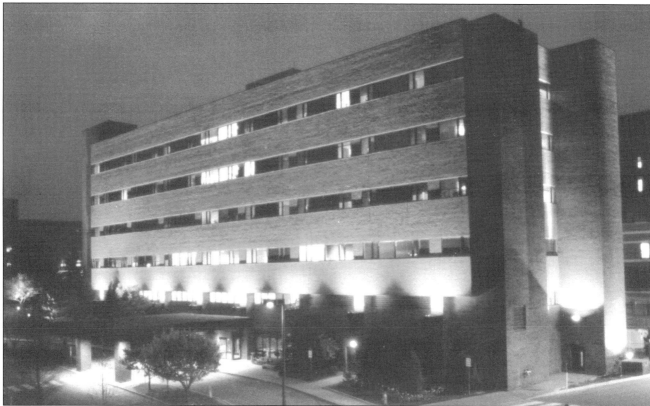

The new main wing of Butler Memorial Hospital. For the first time in its history of expansion, the project did not include new beds, but actually reduced the number of beds—a reflection of the changing face of health care. Spacious lab and x-ray areas were features of the project, as well as renovated patient areas. The accelerated growth of drug and alcohol abuse, lumped together in the term "substance abuse," led to the reassignment of beds to a 20-bed drug and alcohol detoxification and rehabilitation unit.

Courtesy of Butler Memorial Hospital

Today's emergency department treats about 30,000 patients yearly. McCarren said that new doctors who came to BMH's emergency department were continually amazed at the number and variety of the patients they saw.

In the 1980s, the hospital took several important steps in providing service to the community in new ways. The Department of Patient and Community Services was inaugurated, with social workers to help families and patients with such practical problems as obtaining needed equipment, wheelchairs, walkers, etc., as well as providing emotional support. The Education and Training Department began a whole series of in-house education programs for medical staff, and

at the same time initiated a patient education series. In the beginning, the program was a series of videotapes on diabetes; it continued to grow, however, and, in 1995, BMH pioneered a hospital-based Diabetes Management Program to educate diabetics on the proper management of their disease.

Community Education began with a smoking cessation program, working with the National Center for Health Promotion.

That was just the beginning. Today the newly consolidated Education Department provides expectant parent classes, stress management and a host of others. Education also sponsors support groups of all kinds: cancer, chronic fatigue syndrome, arthritis, and others.

Another community service initiated in the eighties was Medic 1. Medic 1 was the vehicle used by the Advanced Life Support Team, on call when sophisticated equipment and training were needed at the scene of an accident. Any county ambulance could call the BMH emergency department in such an emergency, and the team would respond. What was unusual to a community ambulance service of the 1980s was routine to the state-certified paramedics specialized in life-threatening emergencies. The Medic 1 was equipped with EKG monitors, defibrillators, and intravenous fluids, as well as tools designed to rescue someone trapped in a car.

The hospital added other sophisticated services in 1985, including angiography and neurosurgery, and the ICU and CCU (critical care unit) were renovated and upgraded. A year later, laser surgery was introduced.

Butler's sizeable aging population prompted the county commissioners to establish the Area Agency on Aging (outgrowth of a state program) in 1984. The agency operates seniors centers and supplies meals, transportation, legal aid, and many other services to help seniors maintain independence and quality of life as long as possible. Butler Hospital's Priority Care program also targets seniors in the community, offering special health-related and educational services.

Mary Foley (center), long time obstretrical nurse, said, "In 1947 we had only one labor room with four beds, and mothers were transported to the delivery room to give birth. "Today, in our five beautiful birthing suites, mothers can experience labor, delivery and recovery in the same room, with father and/or coach right with her." Courtesy of Butler Memorial Hospital

While much of western Pennsylvania was losing population, Butler County actually reversed the trend. With the improvement of Route 19 and the opening of I-79, Cranberry Township suddenly evolved from quiet little Criders Corners, with its feed store, general store, and gas station, into a full-fledged and affluent suburb with shopping malls and megastores. Cranberry's growth rate— 1,000 new residents per year, fastest in the state and at one time third fastest in the nation—shows no signs of slowing down. With the new families in the area and no health-care services at hand, BMH in 1985 established the Southwest Butler Urgent Care Center.

Strategic Planning

Competition was watchword of the day. Federal and state guidelines for compensation increasingly restricted both inpatient care and length of hospital stay. For some years newspapers and magazines predicted doom due to the spiraling costs of health care; in the eighties it became obvious that the supply of available dollars was shrinking rapidly. The marvelous new technology and advances in health care came at a high price.

At this critical time, BMH initiated a program of strategic planning to continue to supply quality care in a more cost-effective manner. The first step was to find out what the community needed most. They got a partial answer from various statistical studies of county-by-county disease and mortality rates, which showed that heart disease was becoming more of a problem in the county each year. In response, BMH took a significant step in 1988 by opening the cardiopulmonary rehabilitation department to provide important education and a program of controlled exercise to those recovering from heart attacks.

In the late 1980s, Butler Memorial broke new ground with a Total Quality Improvement Process, a familiar tool for corporate America, but new to the healthcare field. A fundamental feature of Total Quality was to look at things in new ways, to determine the causes of problems related to patient care, and to come up with valid strategies for removing or solving the problems. BMH was so successful in building a culture of quality that, when the U.S. government explored the option of expanding the National Malcolm Baldrige Quality Award to health care, it selected Butler as one of only two hospitals in the nation for a site visit to assess how quality can become a part of healthcare delivery.

That the quality improvement process worked is shown by a 1991 patient survey that ranked BMH in the top 16 percent of 400 facilities polled nationwide; 98 percent of Butler County patients polled were happy with their doctors and their hospital care.

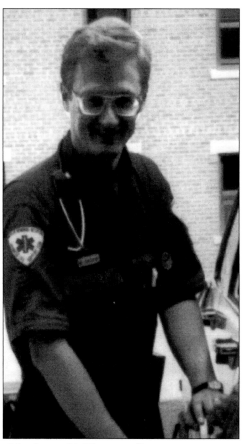

John Spryn, BMH paramedic
Courtesy of Butler Memorial Hospital

Committed to partnering with other agencies and groups as a means of providing better service, BMH, through a joint venture, brought mobile MRI services to the county and then opened its own Breast Imaging Center to provide mammography and education about breast cancer to women.

Butler Hospital has always been committed to providing care for all who need it. In 1989, pregnant women who were uninsured were being bussed an hour away for prenatal care and delivery. The hospital, the board of directors, physicians, and other members of the community met and came up with the Maternal Services Program. Beginning its operation in 1990, the program provides complete and accessible services to mothers, from prenatal care through delivery. In its first few years, the program reduced the incidence of low-birth-weight babies, a prime cause of infant health problems, by 67 percent.

The success of this program led to the question: What happens to the babies after the eight-week follow-up? Once again, BMH worked with all involved—physicians, social workers, community health educators—to develop appropriate care. They gathered information from all the agencies involved with children and from the alumni moms of the Maternal Services Program. This enabled them to design programs and services for these young citizens—to keep them healthy and to provide care when they need it.

Caring Service Meets the Bottom Line

Managed Care in the Nineties

he 1990s brought Butler Memorial Hospital and all its personnel new and important challenges: first and foremost, how to provide quality and caring service in the atmosphere of managed care, which emphasizes the bottom line.

Managed care brought with it a new way of thinking—that the hospital's mission was not just to provide inpatient care, but to play a proactive role in the community's health. Its mission now was to help people stay healthy so that the ever-shrinking supply of health dollars could be spent more effectively.

The changes in health care affected the practice of medicine as well. Twenty years ago most physicians maintained a solo practice; only a few had partners. Today, group practice is becoming the norm. The trend toward specialization in the 1950s and 1960s, and away from family practice, was abruptly reversed with managed care's emphasis on the family or primary care physician as the "gate keeper" in charge of all referrals to specialists. Some members of HMOs have found that their choice of physicians or specialists is limited to "those on the list," although this has changed somewhat in response to complaints from consumers.

Dr. McKee says, "I do have some problems with managed care. I can understand why it came about. When American Automobile Manufacturers found they were spending more on health care than on steel, they realized something had to be done. But the system should not reward doctors for holding down essential costs, such as some tests. That results in bad medicine.

"Nevertheless," he adds. "I do still tell young people to go into medicine. I think it's a fine profession, and most young doctors are idealists as we were. They will have to live with managed care and change it into something we can all live with."

Children And Families First

For years, change and improvements had come piece by piece, but in the nineties the pieces began to fall into place like a jigsaw puzzle.

The 1990s brought new high tech tools: the informational systems provided by computers that link doctors, hospitals, and other community health-care providers so that vital patient information is instantly available when needed. And the first steps into community preventive health in the eighties flowered in the nineties in amazing and gratifying ways.

In 1991, a county program for child victims of sexual abuse, the Parent-Infant Care Center, was threatened with dissolution because of budget cuts. (Juvenile sexual abuse had been a growing problem in the county. In 1988, 70 percent of the substantiated new reports to the County and Youth Services were sexual abuse.) BMH took over the Parent-Infant Care Center and expanded it. The program, now Family Services, provides a family-centered approach, with group treatment for victims, nonoffending parents, and perpetrators. The program works with county Children and Youth Services and has developed a communication network with the county court system and community agencies.

But the hospital did not stop there. Enlisting the cooperation of many agencies concerned with children and families, in 1995 the hospital took over the former armory on North Washington Street and renovated it for a Family First Resource Center. Here many providers of children's services are under one roof and families can obtain help for a whole spectrum of problems, not just sexual abuse. Satellite resource centers were established in Slippery Rock, Moniteau, and Karns City, each with its own community board. The programs supply needed services to children from birth to twelve.

These programs have been possible only

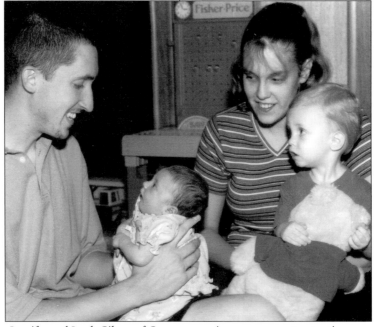

Jennifer and Jacob Gibson of Connoquenessing, very young prospective parents, had no family support. They didn't know who would help. But, as Jennifer explained, "We worked with the Children's Care Program at BMH. They became our support, our family." The BMH Children's Care Program exists for that very purpose. Courtesy of Butler Memorial Hospital

because of widespread community support. The increase in free and below-cost charity services provided by BMH escalated from $500,000 in 1994 to $3.6 million in 1995, largely spent on maternal services and the programs of the Family First Resource Center.

It was concern for the family unit that led the North Main Street Church of God to establish its North Main Street Family Counseling Center, with focus on marriage and the family. The center provides emotional support, counseling, and crisis intervention.

With managed care dictating early release of new mothers—24 to 48 hours for a normal delivery and three to four days for a typical cesarean birth—BMH realized these new mothers needed help. A patient education program helps teach the new moms how to care for their babies, including bathing and breast feeding. But the hospital's concern for mothers and babies begins long before birth—expectant mothers are asked to enroll in the prenatal program as soon as it has been determined they are pregnant. This leads to a healthier pregnancy and a healthier baby. The Caring Angel Program, begun in 1993 as an internal project to raise funds for children's services, is now an important project of the Butler Health System Foundation, charged with the mission of raising money to help pay for a variety of services provided by BMH. In 1997, the program raised $115,000, which the hospital used to buy a sophisticated fetal monitoring system that can, at the touch of a button, offer doctors and nurses important information on the baby before birth. The electronic unit records the mother's contractions and the baby's heartbeat.

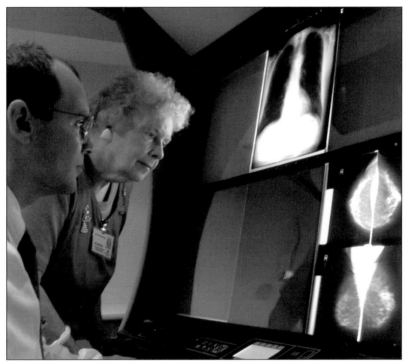

Dr. Bertan Ozgun, radiologist, shows Auxilian Mar-Bet Cavanaugh how the Smartlight technology works. The Smartlight enhances images on x-ray, focusing in on problem areas and enlarging them at the touch of a finger, making breast cancers or masses much easier to detect than on the conventional viewer. BMH is one of only a few hospitals in Pennsylvania to have such a machine that can help detect breast cancer much earlier and, consequently, help to save more lives.

Courtesy of Butler Memorial Hospital

"The alarm is not audible to the patient, which might add to the mother's distress. Instead it appears on the system. If, for example, the baby's heart rate drops, that information will immediately flash on the screen. The nurse or doctor, wherever they are, will be able to see it and respond," she adds. The maternity unit staff has had special training sessions in operating the system and is linked with the OB/GYN doctors affiliated with the hospital.

"If any emergency would arise, we can see it immediately and respond promptly. The system allows us to monitor a patient even from our office or home and respond quickly to any event," says Dr. Philip Lenko, of Advanced OB/GYN Associates. Each of the five birthing suites, the birthing suite exam room, and even some patient rooms in the maternity unit have a system hookup, with monitors linked to a central unit that allows a constant stream of information. Doctors and nurses can be in another area, yet still keep tabs on how the patient's labor is progressing.

"The system has a built-in alarm that notifies the nurse or doctor the second something goes wrong," says Ann Snodgrass, director of maternal services.

From Babies to Seniors

In direct response to the current trend of discharging patients sooner rather than later, in 1991 the hospital established the Transitional Care Facility. This unit, which originally had nineteen beds, has recently been increased to twenty-five and moved to the north wing, in an attractive and more homelike setting. It provides skilled nursing care for patients who have been in the hospital and are ready for discharge, but are not yet ready to go home. While they are in this wing they are under medical supervision, a welcome feature for both patients and concerned families.

Opened in 1992, the cardiac catheterization lab provides vital diagnostic services that patients could previously only get in Pittsburgh. Clair Hutzler of Butler appreciated this improvement. He had gone to BMH in the early nineties with severe chest pains. Diagnosed with heart trouble, he was sent to Pittsburgh for heart catheterization and, subsequently, balloon angioplasty.

Hutzler said, "After the procedure I started on a monitored program of cardiac rehab exercise at Butler Memorial. Twelve weeks after that, I began a maintenance exercise program three days a week. . . . But then my wife died in February of '96 and I was really under a lot of stress." Soon he needed another catheterization, but this time he could have it done in BMH's cardiac cath lab. "It meant a lot to me to stay in the community," he said. "I got really good care and now I'm back on exercise maintenance in cardiac rehab at BMH."

The hospital helped Hutzler make changes in his diet as well. "The dietician at Butler Memorial taught me a lot about how diet affects my heart," he said. "I used to eat a lot of meat and I would just grab anything in a hurry. And I have a real sweet tooth. Now I look at labels for low-fat foods and eat far less meat, ice cream, and chocolates. I feel a lot better, and I know I'm healthier."

An important move in bringing health care to all parts of the county was the creation of Butler Medical Associates as an extension of the hospital in 1992. BMA, a multiphysician practice specializing in family and general internal medicine, today brings quality medical care to parts of the county through its Saxonburg, Chicora and Butler offices. The hospital has also developed outpatient laboratory and x-ray testing sites in several locations throughout Butler County.

In 1993, the hospital opened the Pain Management Center, the only center in a twenty-five-mile radius to treat chronic pain. In addition, it initiated a geriatric psychiatry program, and the following year, opened the Sleep Center for those afflicted with sleep apnea and other sleep disorders.

Another partnership is that of BMH and the state health department in a pilot program now operating in the county called the Community Health Network. The state health office in Butler is now closed and BMH has taken the services formerly provided by the state to every section of the county: immunization clinics for children and for those traveling in areas where special immunizations are needed; three testing clinics, one for TB, one for AIDS, and one for sexually transmitted diseases.

A big advantage for Butler County residents is the convenience of the new setup; instead of one office centrally located, BMH takes the services to every part of the county on a rotating basis. The state still manages any epidemics that occur, from head lice in a school to an outbreak of salmonella or other disease. The basis for the pilot is the belief that those who are directly involved in health care can provide the services more efficiently and cost-effectively.

One of the most recent and exciting partnerships is the one the hospital entered into with the Veterans Administration Medical Center. Together they share a state-of-the-art scanner with a computerized tomography system that can provide vastly improved diagnostic services to patients. The scanner, which was purchased by the medical center, is housed at Butler Hospital, since the hospital has the staff and facilities to maintain the new equipment. In return, veterans have access to the new machine whenever medical center doctors request it and, of course, the center will not pay for its use. This is what both administrations see as the first of many possible joint ventures between the two medical institutions.

Community Health Planning

A tremendous accomplishment of the decade was the establishment in 1994 of the Butler Health Advisory Council, a community-based health planning team. Such a team of community leaders could not even have existed in 1990, when health-care reform and managed care, although a reality elsewhere, were just beginning in Butler County. The reality of fewer dollars brought home to everyone the need to eliminate costly duplication of services and work together to make sure that every necessary service is provided in the most cost effective way. The providers' focus had shifted from a narrow competitive stance to a cooperative community orientation.

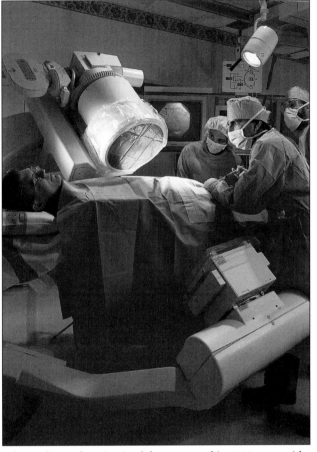

The cardiac catheterization lab was opened in 1992, to provide vital diagnostic services for patients who previously had to go to Pittsburgh. This procedure— performed on patients who, physicians think may be at risk of heart attack, on patients following cardiac surgery, or to assess damage on someone who has a heart attack—helps determine the appropriate treatment.
Courtesy of Butler Memorial Hospital

task was to conduct a thorough community health assessment and gauge community health priorities. This assessment describes in detail what the major health issues are—some of them unique to Butler County—and also describes those issues that are specific to certain areas of the county. For example, while cardiac disease is a problem in all of Butler County, the southwest and southeast areas have the highest mortality. On the other hand, there is a higher rate of diabetes in central Butler County than in other areas.

The council developed eleven task forces, which began presenting reports and recommendations in 1996. Interestingly, although people cited a number of problems—including geriatric health issues—

The council's purpose was to identify the community's most pressing health problems and assist BMH to develop action plans. The council recognized that community health is not just going to the doctor or the hospital, but strengthening the family, making sure everyone has access to primary care, and providing education for a healthy lifestyle.

Butler County was one of the first communities in the country to create a community health plan and take active and positive steps to implement it. The first

their main concern was not knowing what kind of help was available and how to access it. That led to the Community Information Resource Line, a "hotline" that provides information about services by phone or Internet, twenty-four hours a day, seven days a week. A database was set up to allow a caseworker or agency person to print out relevant information.

Many hospitals nationally had created voluminous documents similar to Butler Hospital's Community Health Assessment. However, most of them gathered dust on shelves, instead of using them as Butler Hospital has done, to create a care system tailored to community needs.

Still a Community Hospital

Entering the Twenty-first Century with the HeartCenter

Targeted as the number one concern in Butler, cardiac disease has taken its toll, often because patients did not survive the trip to Pittsburgh. According to the hospital's Community Health Assessment, Butler County and the surrounding communities had a higher death rate from heart disease than the state of Pennsylvania and even the nation as a whole. The distances people had to travel for open heart surgery was an important factor in the equation.

As the hospital addressed this concern, many questions arose: Could BMH establish a first-class cardiac center in Butler? How would it be staffed?

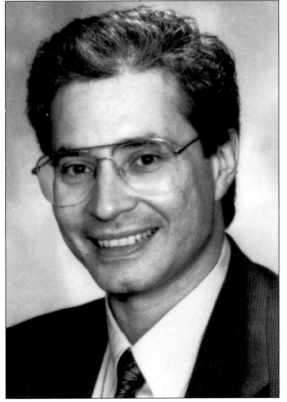

Dr. George Davliakos, first surgeon and medical director in the open heart program at BMH's HeartCenter
Courtesy of Butler Memorial Hospital

Who would perform the sophisticated surgery required? And how would the post-operative patients be cared for?

The questions were answered for the community on March 11, 1998, when BMH President Joseph A. Stewart announced the opening of the hospital's Heart-Center, scheduled for July 1, and the selection of Three Rivers Cardiac Institute in Carnegie to help develop the new heart surgery program.

"We have chosen to remain dedicated to this community as an independent hospital, but at the same time we vowed to bring the best clinical services to this hospital," said President Stewart. "We have done just that with our Heart-Center by bringing in Three Rivers Cardiac Institute, conducting our staff training for the HeartCenter at Mercy Hospital, and by partnering with the same cardiac anesthesiology team used at

Allegheny Genera Hospital. Together we are committed to developing a first-rate program here at BMH."

Headed by Ronald V. Pellegrini, M.D., well known heart surgeon, Three Rivers Cardiac Institute currently performs heart surgery at the University of Pittsburgh Medical Center, Mercy Hospital, UPMC Passavant, and Washington Hospital—and now, at Butler Hospital. Three Rivers includes some of the finest surgeons in the country, including Dr. George P. Davliakos, who serves as the medical director for open heart surgery at Butler's HeartCenter.

According to Dr. Davliakos, he is pleased to be a resident of Butler and to have the chance to work with the local cardiologists in developing the HeartCenter. "We had the opportunity at the HeartCenter to obtain results that are as good as, and even better than the national standards by eliminating the inefficiencies that exist in other hospitals and because of the quality of care that already exists at Butler Hospital," he said.

The hospital has also added angioplasty to its cardiac services. Angioplasty, the insertion of a balloon-tipped catheter to widen the coronary arteries, can reduce the need for bypass surgery by 80 percent.

Meanwhile, Dr. Davliakos is delighted with the progress the HeartCenter has made in a short time. "The results have been as good or better than in Pittsburgh hospitals."

Statistics show that the key to successful treatment of heart disease is to begin within the "golden hour," before heart muscle damage becomes permanent. According to analysts, the Butler community has had some 200 excess deaths from heart attacks yearly, lives that perhaps could have been saved had treatment been received in timely fashion. With the addition of the full spectrum of cardiac services, including cardiovascular screenings, cardiac rehabilitation, a chest pain clinic to provide patients with a fast track to service, a public education program to teach early recognition of cardiac symptoms, cardiac catheterization, angioplasty, and now cardiac surgery, many of these unnecessary deaths can be avoided.

By November of 1999 the team had performed more than 300 open heart surgeries, with statistics that met and even exceeded the national standards. The volume was such that the hospital needed to expand the HeartCenter, adding new recovery and private waiting rooms, redesigning the cardiac rehabilitation area, renovating the cardiac ultrasound and peripheral vascular laboratory, as well as adding a second cardiac catheterization laboratory. A second cardiac surgeon came on board as well as vascular (vein) surgeons.

The HeartCenter has proved a winner: patients are enthusiastic and pleased with the care. They appreciate the opportunity to stay in familiar surroundings with their own cardiologists to see them post-operatively. An added plus: no long drives or parking problems for their families!

Cancer and The Women's Imaging Center

With the HeartCenter up and running successfully, it was time to address Butler County's second greatest health concern: cancer. For women, breast cancer is the number one killer in Butler County as well as nationally. This statistic provided a special, and encouraging, challenge, since breast cancer is one of the most treatable malignancies if detected early enough. Essential to early detection are regular self-examinations and regular mammography.

The Community Health Assessment determined that for Butler County women aged 50 and over, for whom yearly mammograms are recommended, only 55.3% complied, lower even than the region's 61%. Although for both groups 100% would be ideal, these figures were certainly much too low and offered the possibility for great improvement.

A cancer task force, formed by the Community Advisory Council, decided that the first preventive focus should be breast cancer awareness. They identified the most at-risk areas of the county and have trained volunteers from those areas to educate people on breast health awareness.

While these programs were getting underway, the hospital made a major commitment to women's health, with the opening of the Women's Imaging Center in the summer of 1999. The Center offers women privacy and the convenience of "one-stop-shopping;" no longer must women go through outpatient registration and the general x-ray area for mammography and other tests. Registration and all women's diagnostic services are available in this attractive, patient-friendly unit, where the finest, most up-to-date equipment has been installed, to give women the latest in advanced diagnostic care. A special feature of the unit is the Smartlight Digital Film Viewer, a vastly impro-ved version of the lightbox radiologists use to exam-

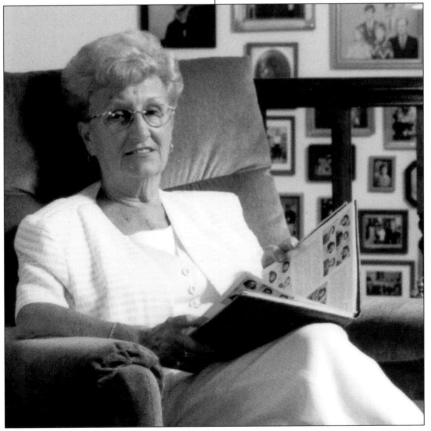

Alison Guthrie Jones became the first patient to undergo bypass surgery at the new BMH HeartCenter. She was glad that she was able to receive this service close to home.
Courtesy of Butler Memorial Hospital

ine film, contributed by the BMH Women's Auxiliary, which can help pinpoint & diagnose cancers much earlier when they are most treatable.

The hospital has also set up satellite outpatient mammography units in Slippery Rock and the Butler Mall to provide more convenient service for women in those areas.

A Pilot Program For Stroke Victims

Stroke in Butler County is also a major concern, especially for county residents age 48-64—young for strokes. BMH, in partnership with the University of Pittsburgh Medical Center, is providing state-of-the-art treatment for stroke patients in Butler Hospital. Immediate treatment is vital to a patient's recovery, since there is only a three hour window of opportunity—that is, the period in which such special treatment is effective.

Not long ago, it was believed that nothing much could be done to help someone who suffered a stroke. Now, medicine has learned that aggressive, prompt treatment can greatly alleviate the effects and more complete recovery can be attained.

A Community Hospital – Still

In November 1997, BMH held a reception and display of hospital and medical history to kick off the celebration of its 100th anniversary. The high point of the featured program was the announcement by the president, Joseph Stewart, that Butler Memorial Hospital would remain an independent community hospital—partnering with others when necessary or desirable. It would not become a cog in one of the mega-hospital machines, but would continue to work with all local health care providers to fulfill the needs of the Butler County community. This meant that the community itself—not some giant bureaucracy—could continue to determine what it needed—and how to provide it.

Butler Memorial Hospital, an integral part of the Butler Health System, remains Butler County's, created and maintained by volunteer efforts—volunteers that come from every area and population segment. The Auxiliary, the Candystripers and the Red Cross volunteers have given hundreds of thousands of hours of service. They work in almost every area of the hospital, where they provide escort service, help and support to families, as well as assistance to hospital employees in almost every department. Through its Cherry Tree Gift Shop and Hostess Shoppe, as well as other fundraising activities, the Auxiliary has given the hospital over $1.5 million dollars through the years, enabling it to buy much-needed and expensive life-saving equipment.

The Board of Directors, the Health System Foundation Board and other volunteers have helped to raise the money to support the hospital and extend its preventive and charitable care—not only in its important daily operation, but in new programs that reach into the community in all areas of the county.

And, most important, the community has supported the hospital through the years—financially and in other ways.

In the end, a great strength of an excellent community hospital is its compassionate, human—and humane—care for its patients. Butler Memorial Hospital's patients are people, not numbers or abstract notes on a chart. All hospitals have to struggle to keep the personal touch today when economics dictates fewer resources, more paper work, shorter hospital stays and more expensive high tech machines. Fortunately, providing unsurpassed care is at the heart of BMH. It is its vision. It is its commitment. It is its very definition.

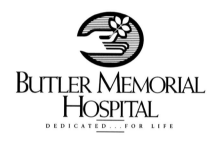

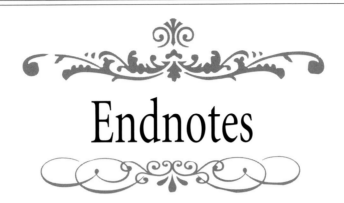

Endnotes

Chapter One

(1) Brackenridge, H.M., *Recollections of the West*

(2) Diller, Theodore, M.D., *Pioneer Medicine in Western Pennsylvania*

(3) Knoedler, Christine, *The Harmony Society, a 19th Century American Utopia*

(4) Ruch, Shelby Miller, *Windows on the Past, A Look Back at 19th Century Life in Zelienople and Harmony, Pennsylvania*

(5) Ibid.

(6) McKee, James, *Twentieth Century History of Butler and Butler County, Pa., and Representative Citizens*

(7) Negley, John H., *Butler Sentinel* "Recollections"

(8) Brown, R.C., "*Butler County, Pennsylvania*"

(9) Ibid.

(10) Ibid.

(11) *Butler Sentinel*, January 1890

(12) McKee, James *Twentieth Century History of Butler and Butler County, Pa., and Representative Citizens*

(13) *The Butler Eagle*

(14) McKee, James *Twentieth Century History of Butler and Butler County, Pa., and Representative Citizens*

(15) Ibid.

Chapter Two

(16) Ibid.

(17) *The Butler County Citizen*

(18) *Butler Centennial Souvenir, 1900*

(19) Nurses had first been used in a large scale in this country during the Civil War, when mothers, sisters, and daughters wanted to help care for their men in uniform.

(20) *The Butler Eagle*

Chapter Three

(21) In the United States in 1900 there were more than 30 deaths per 100,000 population.

(22) *The Butler Eagle*, November 7, 1903

(23) McKee, James T*wentieth Century History of Butler and Butler County, Pa., and Representative Citizens*

(24) *The Millerstown Herald*, July, 1900

Chapter Four

(25) *The Butler Eagle*, October, 1907

(26) Ibid.

(27) Baycura, Peter, Lyndora Chronicles: *The Legendary Decades 1902-1921*

Chapter Five

(28) *Time*, February 23, 1918

(29) *The Butler Eagle*, August 1918

(30) *The Daily Citizen*, September 23,1918

(31) *The Butler Eagle*, October 5, 1918

(32) Garrett, Kelly, *The Butler Eagle* , October 18, 1998

Chapter Six

(33) Kuhn, Leroy, It Was Yesterday, Edited by Mechling Associates, Inc., printed by Closson Press

(34) *The Butler Eagle*, 1925

(35) *The Butler Eagle*, February, 1925

Chapter Ten

(36) The Hospital Association was an organization of Butler County citizens responsible for electing BMH's board of directors. Anyone could join for a membership fee of $10.00.

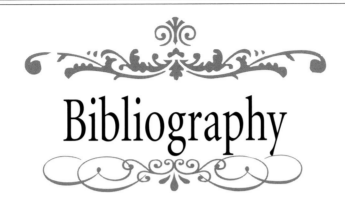

Bibliography

American History Desk Reference, A Stonesong Press Book, New York: MacMillan USA, 1997.

Armstrong, David, and Armstrong, Elizabeth Metzger. *The Great American Medicine Show.* New York: Prentice Hall, 1991

Arndt, Karl J.R., *George Rapp's Harmony Society 1705-1847*, revised edition. Associated University Presses, Inc.,

Baycura, Peter, *Lyndora Chronicles: The Legendary Decades 1902-1921*, Butler, Pennsylvania: John Franklin Baycura, 1998.

Brown, R.C., ed., *Butler County, Pennsylvania*, N.P.; R.C.Brown, 1895.

Butler Centennial Souvenir, Butler, PA: Godwin & Curry, 1900

Butler County Pennsylvania 1800-1950, Official Sesquicentennial Book, Butler, Pennsylvania: Baycura Publishing, 1950.

Diller, Theodore, M.D., *Pioneer Medicine in Western Pennsylvania*, New York: Paul B. Hoeber, Inc., 1987

Duffy, John, *The Healers: The Rise of the Medical Establishment*, New York: McGraw-Hill, 1976.

Dunlop, Richard, *Doctors of the American Frontier*, Garden City, New York: Doubleday & Co., Inc., 1965.

Goldinger, Ralph, and Fetters, Audrey, *Butler County, the Second Hundred Years*, N.P. (no date given)

Gordon, Maurice Bear, M.D., *Aesculapius Comes to the Colonies*, Ventor, New Jersey: Ventnor Publishers, Inc., 1949.

HealthScene, Butler Memorial Hospital

History of Butler County, Pennsylvania 1796-1883, Chicago: Waterman Watkins & Co., 1883

Knoedler, Christine, *The Harmony Society, a 19th Century American Utopia*, New York: Vantage Inc., 1954.

Marks, Geoffrey, and Beatty, William K., *Women in White*, New York: Charles Scribner's Sons, 1972

McKee, James A., *Twentieth Century History of Butler and Butler County, Pa., and Representative Citizens*, Chicago: Richman Arnold, 1909.

Pitzer, Donald E., ed., *George Rapp's Disciples, Pioneers and Heirs: A Registry of the Harmonists in America,* compiled with an introduction by Karl J.R. Arndt, LeighAnn Chamness, Evansville, Indiana: University of Southern Indiana Press, 1992.

Pozar, Stephen M., and Purvis, Jean B., *Butler, A Pictorial History,* revised edition, Virginia Beach, Virginia: Donning Company Publishers, 1994.

Prizm, Butler Memorial Hospital

Ruch, Shelby Miller, *Windows on the Past, A Look Back at 19th Century Life in Zelienople and Harmony, Pennsylvania, 1998.* A collection of the author's articles from *The News Weekly.*

The White Sheet, Butler Memorial Hospital

NEWSPAPERS

Butler County Sentinel

The Millerstown Herald

The Butler Citizen

The Union Herald

The Daily Citizen

The Butler Eagle